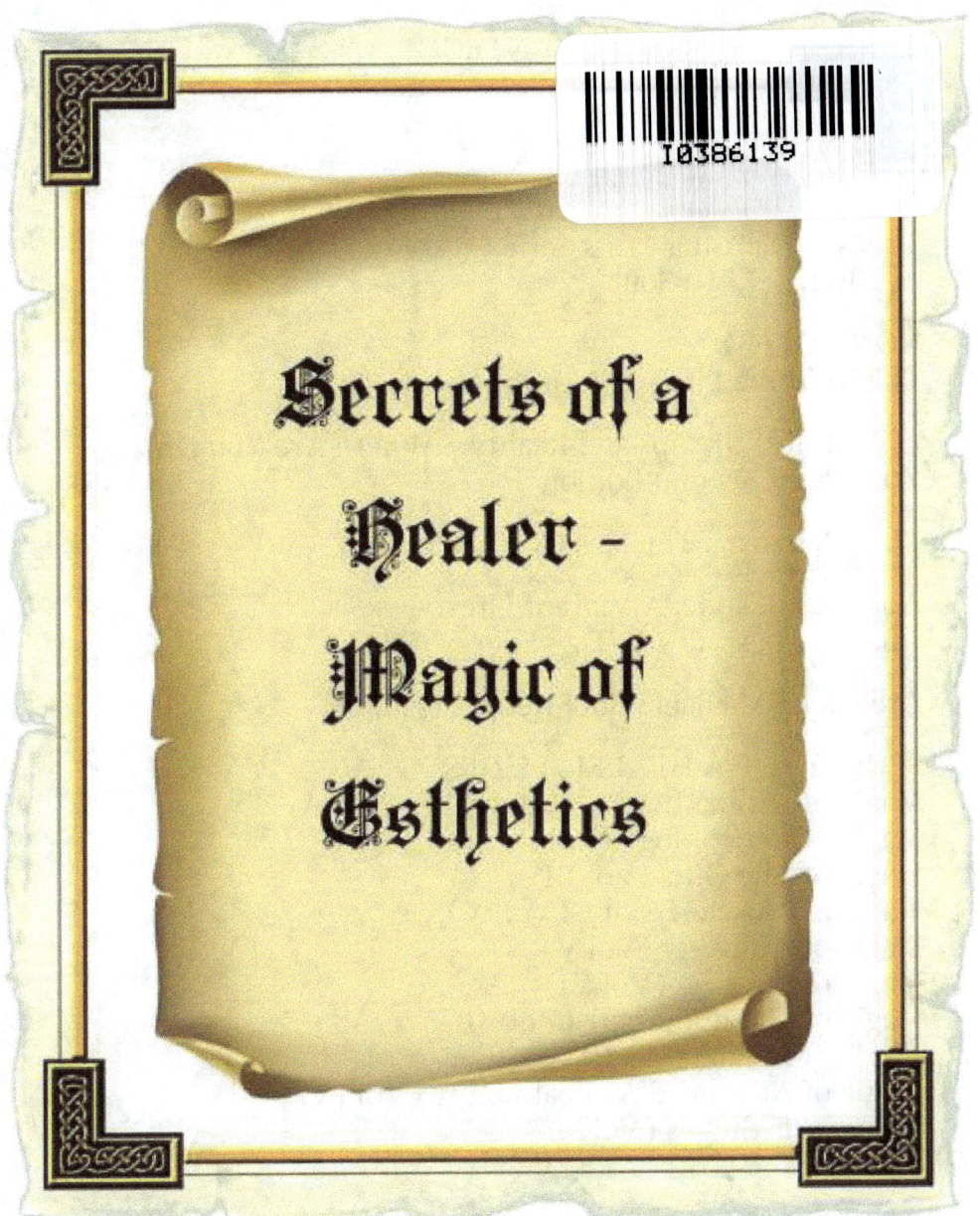

ALSO BY CONSTANCE SANTEGO

FICTION
(Novels are based on actual events)
The Nine Spiritual Gifts Series:
    Journey of a Soul

NONFICTION
The Intuitive Life – Gift of Prophecy

Fairy Tales, Dreams and Reality... Where Are You On Your Path? Second Edition

Your Persona... The Mask You Wear

Angelic Lifestyle, A Vibrant Lifestyle & Angelic Lifestyle's 42-Day Energy Cleanse

Archangel Michael's Soul Retrieval Guide

SECRETS OF A HEALER, SERIES:
Magic of Aromatherapy (Vol I)
Magic of Reflexology (Vol II)
Magic of The Gifts (Vol III)
Magic of Muscle Testing (Vol IV)
Magic of Iridology (Vol V)
Magic of Massage (Vol VI)
Magic of Hypnotherapy (Vol VII)
Magic of Reiki (Vol VIII)
Magic of Advanced Aromatherapy (Vol IX)
Magic of Esthetics (Vol X)

SECRETS OF A HEALER

VOL. X
MAGIC OF ESTHETICS

Constance Santego

Maximillian Enterprises
Kelowna, BC

Secrets Of A Healer – Magic of Esthetics
Copyright © 2020 by Constance Santego.

All rights reserved. No part of this publication may be reproduced, distributed or transmitted in any form or by any means, including photocopying, recording, or other electronic or mechanical methods, without the prior written permission of the publisher, except in the case of brief quotations embodied in critical reviews and certain other noncommercial uses permitted by copyright law. For permission requests, write to the publisher, addressed "Attention: Permissions Coordinator," at the address below.

Copy Editor and Interior Design: Constance Santego
Book Layout: ©2017 BookDesignTemplates.com
Cover Design: Jennifer Louie

Ordering Information:
Quantity sales. Special discounts are available on quantity purchases by corporations, associations, and others. For details, contact the "Special Sales Department" at the address above.

Trade paperback ISBN: 978-1-7772220-6-2
Created and published In Canada. Printed and bound in the United States of America

First Edition
Published by Maximillian Enterprises
Kelowna, BC
Canada
www.constancesantego.ca

Dedication
To all the wonderful people who not only make you look beautiful but make you feel that way too.

Preventative medicine starts with self-care!

–Constance Santego

Contents

Preface viii
Note to Reader ix
Learning Outcome x
What is Esthetics? 1
    Traditional Spa 2
    History 2
    Esthetician vs. Day Spa Practitioner 6
Spa Regulations and Safety 8
    First Aid 16
    Sanitization Rules 17
Spa Techniques 23
    Mani's 24
    Pedi's 49
    Facials 61
    Make-Up 115
    Eyelash & Eyebrow Tinting 144
    Waxing 150
    Body Polish/Scrub 162
    Bronzing 165
    Back Treatments 168
    Body Wraps 170
What Makes A Great Practitioner? 212
Client Consultation 222
Bibliography 224
Message From The Author 227

Preface

The Miracle of Esthetics

I did not find Esthetics, it found me. My daughter wanted to go to College for Esthetics, and it was cheaper for me to bring the courses into my college than it was to send her to school. And voila, my college offered an Esthetics Diploma.

Of course, I then had to take all the classes myself. And years later started to teach the subject matter, while owning many Spas over the years.

I still remember my first mani-care, I was in Heaven, it was so peaceful and relaxing. That was the moment that I realized that these pampering modalities were therapeutic. I decided that moment to love them as much as my healing modalities because that is what they were, preventative medicine techniques!

Note to Reader

Esthetics is not intended to replace traditional medicine. Persons with physical problems should ALWAYS seek the service of a professional doctor.

Your Doctor still plays a vital role in your health care. If I break my leg, I will need a Doctor and all the nurses and staff that work in the Hospital.

My understanding of Integrated Medicine is that we play a significant role in taking care of our health. What we put into our bodies, how hard we work our bodies, the stress level we allow into our everyday life, and the positive or negative energy we attract around us all play a role in our wellbeing.

Shift happens...Create magic!

Learning Outcome

When you have completed this book and studied the concepts and techniques, you will be able to perform basic Spa techniques to help reduce stress and beautify your body, mind, and soul. For you, your friends, and family to enjoy.

- You will learn many spa treatments and how to incorporate them without the use of water.
- You will learn about many modalities, techniques, and recipes of natural ingredients that you can use and promote wellness and your overall wellbeing.

What is Esthetics?

AKA Aesthetics.
Esthetics means:
- of, relating to, or dealing with aesthetics or the beautiful.
- Pleasing in appearance.
- Done or made to improve a person's appearance or to correct defects in a person's appearance.

Originally the word or definition of 'SPA' meant a type of water therapy, but today, very few will offer water treatments. Most Spas today are considered 'Dry Spas.'

Spas (wet spa), Day Spas, and private spa establishments have been around in one way or another for centuries. Cleopatra is incredibly famous for how she wore make-up on her eyes. In the last twenty years, North America has had a huge increase in the demand for spa and dry spa treatments.

Spa treatments are not only for the rich and famous anymore. Teenagers, as well as ladies well into their eighties, love having their nails done.

Traditional Spa

Thalassotherapy
Thalassotherapy is a Greek word used to refer to spa treatments that employ seawater and algae marine extracts. Perhaps you think of salty water as drying, but these treatments are excellent for dry skin and cellulite. Algae marine extracts also increase circulation, thus helping to firm the skin and reduce fat accumulation.

Balneotherapy
Balneotherapy is the marine treatment of crystals and properties from the sea in a hydrotherapy tub. Enjoying an invigorating underwater massage while the properties nourish and rejuvenate the body.

History

The Turkish Bath

Let us begin with a little bit about Turkish baths. The Definition of a Turkish Bath is, a type of bath in which the bather sweats freely in a room which is heated by a continuous flow of hot, dry air (or in two or three such rooms with hotter temperatures) followed by a full-body wash (sometimes preceded by a cold plunge), then by a massage, and finally a period of relaxation in a cooling room.

It is the dryness of air that distinguishes the Victorian Turkish bath from other types- the vapor bath, the Russian steam bath, or the Finnish Sauna (in the last of which, water is periodically ladled onto the stove or heat source, so as to dampen an otherwise totally dry heat source). The dryness of the air in the Victorian Turkish bath also, perhaps surprisingly distinguishes it from the Turkish baths and hammams which are still to be found in Turkey today.

Turkey in the nineteenth century were many baths or hammams to be found, not just in Turkey, but right across the Middle East generally. Many can still be found but their number is decreasing. What we call the Turkish bath was really a re-invention of the Roman bath, which was invented in 1856 (most recently); such baths to this day are frequently known on the European continent, the most famous perhaps being, Friedrichsbad at Baden-Baden, Germany.

The oldest known spa (Mineral bath) still in existence is in Merano, Italy, where there is evidence of organized use of the spring dating back 5,000 years ago. It is quite possible the wandering humanoids may have soaked their tired feet in the spring. Some historians feel this could have been even later than 5,000 years ago.

It is thought that the Egyptians used baths for therapeutic purposes as early as 2000 BC. Evidence of actual spa construction also exists from the Pharaohs, King of Media, in 600 BC. The earliest forms of hot tubs were simply a caldera in which sizzling stones had to be placed to heat the water. From the early time, our ancestors enjoyed the benefits of natural hot water springs, and thus, hydrotherapy was born!

THE GREEKS

Mineral and thermal baths showed up later in history around 500 B.C. in Greece. The early Greek baths were built near natural hot springs and volcanoes.

Greek celebrities and the elite would meet at these hot springs to exchange philosophical views and treat physical ailments. Plato considered anyone who did not know how to swim to be uneducated. Hippocrates, (460-375 B.C) believed to be the founder of Medicine, recommended hydrotherapy to treat disorders such as jaundice and rheumatism.

THE ROMANS

The Romans also enjoyed mineral waters, but the ancient Roman baths were more recreational areas used by hundreds of citizens at the same time as opposed to personal hygiene and aquatic therapy.

Stone tubs were serviced by elaborate aqueduct systems carrying mineral water throughout complex private rooms, steam rooms, and private baths. The largest of all Roman baths was the Diocletian, completed in AD 305, it covered an area of 130,000 square yards.

Romans were the first to go to the unctuarium where they had servants rub oil onto their skin. Next, they would move to a tepidarium or warm room where they would lie around chatting. From there, it was on to the hot and steamy caldarium, similar to a Turkish bath. Here they sat and perspired, scraping their skin with a curved metal tool known as a strigil. After a dip in the caldarium (hot bath), they would take a quick dip in a frigidarium (cold bath).

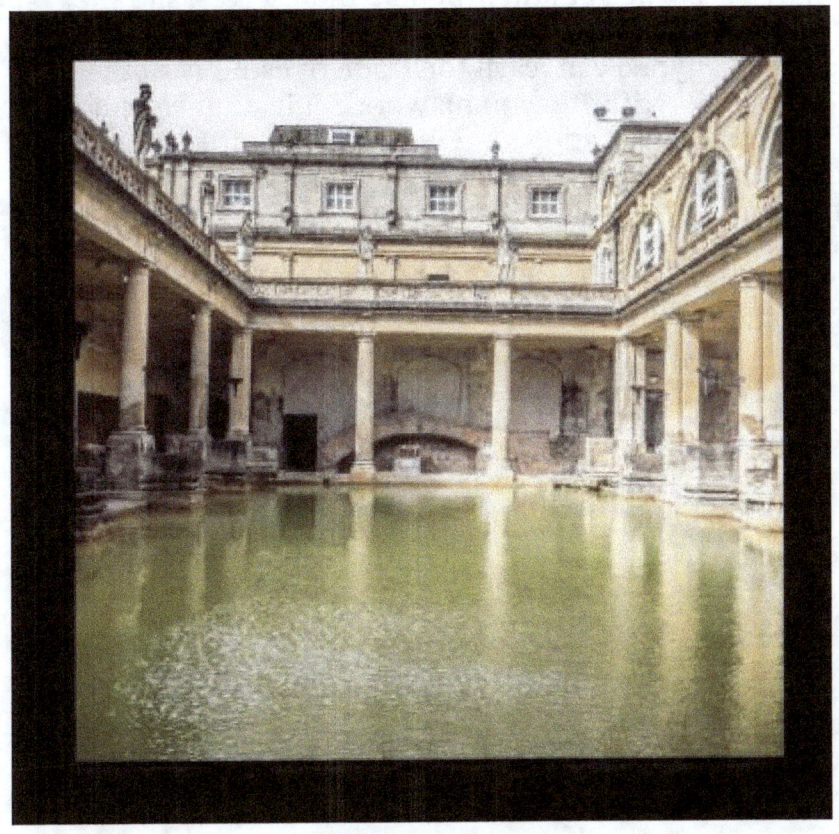

Esthetician vs. Day Spa Practitioner

An Esthetician has graduated from a program and has received a diploma. The practitioner may use all the tools taught and can manipulate the tissue of the body.

A Spa Practitioner has also graduated from a program and has received a diploma but may not use metal tools or manipulated the body. They are beautifying the body using pampering techniques.

Many Spas will train their people themselves, and the practitioner has no certificate. Legally, at the moment in Canada, anyone can learn the trade of esthetics, but without a certificate, you may not get insurance or a business license, and you will have difficulties joining any associations. You will be okay working for someone else but not for yourself.

What you will be learning in this book is what I taught my students... nothing saying you can't work on yourself.

What I taught my Estheticians
- Mani-care
- Manicure
- Pedi-care
- Pedicure
- Spa Facial (no extractions)
- Advanced Facials (with extractions and machines)
- Back Treatments (facial for the back)
- Body wraps
- Body Scrubs and Polish
- Massage
- Reflexology
- Aromatherapy
- Energy Balancing (similar to Reiki)
- Waxing
- Lash & Brow Tinting
- Make-up
- Anatomy, pathology, and business

Artificial Nails (gel or Acrylic) was another program that could be added to the Esthetician program

Spa Regulations and Safety

In Canada, health regulations are the jurisdiction of each province where Ministries of Health enact guidelines, undertake inspections, and provide education to help salon establishments eliminate or mitigate the effects of communicable disease.

Personal Hygiene
(A well done up person makes more money! Proven fact)
Hair, Hands, clothes, breath, body smells, and perspiration. It is also a proven fact that people like to do business with people who are well-groomed and clean.

Leading Spas of Canada

On July 21, 2010, National Program Assesses Safety & Hygiene Standards in Spas standards were set...

Leading Spas of Canada (LSC) has introduced the Quality Assurance Program to provide consistent standards for safety, hygiene, and business standards for the Canadian spa industry, offering reassurance and uncompromising quality for spa guests.

This extensive program was developed by Leading Spas of Canada's Standards & Practices Committee and is based on the rigorous standards supported by all member spas. The Quality Assurance program includes on-site assessments by third-party evaluators to ensure all the standards are met or exceeded.

Upon completing the assessment and meeting or exceeding all standards, the spas receive a certificate and seal of approval for display on-site and in marketing materials, recognizing their Quality Assurance status. The QAA icon serves as a visual indicator for spa guests and staff of the spa's commitment to safety and hygiene standards.

While several 'ratings' programs exist which grade, spas based on the amenities available, the Quality Assurance verification process culminates in a strict pass or fail. Spa offerings and amenities vary dramatically and at the heart of this program is not to measure the value of amenities or size of the spa, but the desire to ensure all spas meet essential safety, hygiene and operational standards, offering confidence and comfort to the spa management, employees and the guest.

The Law in Canada

Ergonomics - *Work Safe BC*
Protecting ourselves from health hazards at work
- *Massage Table height (back issues)*
- *Aromatherapy essential oil overdose (toxins)*
- *Reflexology; our thumbs (joint issues)*
- *Massage; our wrists (joint issues)*
- *Open cuts (we have on our hands or fingers – and if a client has any on any part of the skin we touch – cross-contamination could happen)*
- *Touching a client then touching our own face (rubbing an itchy nose for an example)*

Canada is extremely strict on its health regulations; the health and welfare of Canadians is a priority. Pathogens in the spa industry are regulated very closely.

What is a pathogen?
- Viral - herpes
- Bacteria - cold
- Fungal -warts
- Parasites - bugs

A pathogen or infectious agent - in colloquial terms, a germ — is a microbe or microorganism such as a virus, bacterium, prion, or fungus that causes disease in its animal or plant host. There are several substrates, including pathways whereby pathogens can invade a host; the principal pathways have different episodic time frames, but soil contamination has the longest or most persistent potential for harboring a pathogen.

The body contains many natural orders of defense against some of the common pathogens (such as Pneumocystis) in the form of the human immune system and by some "helpful" bacteria present in the human body's normal flora. However, if the immune system or "good" bacteria is damaged in any way (such as by chemotherapy, human immunodeficiency virus (HIV), or antibiotics being taken to kill other pathogens), pathogenic bacteria that were being held at bay can proliferate and cause harm to the host. Such cases are called opportunistic infections.

Types of pathogens

Following is a listing of different types of notable pathogens as categorized by their structural characteristics and some of the known effects.

Pathogen, Examples, and Typical effects

BACTERIA

Escherichia coli	honeymoon cystitis or urinary tract infection (UTI), peritonitis, foodborne illness
Mycobacterium tuberculosis	tuberculosis
Bacillus anthracis	anthrax
Salmonella	foodborne illness
Staphylococcus aureus	toxic shock syndrome
Streptococcus pneumoniae	pneumonia
Streptococcus pyogenes	strep throat
Helicobacter pylori	Stomach ulcers
Francisella tularensis	tularemia

VIRUSES

Hepatitis A, B, C, D and E	liver disease
Influenza virus	flu
Herpes simplex	virus herpes
Molluscum contagiosum	rash
Human immunodeficiency virus	AIDS

Human Coronavirus Types
Coronaviruses are named for the crown-like spikes on their surface. The seven coronaviruses that can infect people are:
Common human coronaviruses
1. 229E (alpha coronavirus)
2. NL63 (alpha coronavirus)
3. OC43 (beta coronavirus)
4. HKU1 (beta coronavirus)

Other human coronaviruses
    5. MERS-CoV (the beta coronavirus that causes Middle East Respiratory Syndrome, or MERS)
    6. SARS-CoV (the beta coronavirus that causes a severe acute respiratory syndrome, or SARS)
    7. **SARS-CoV-2 (the novel coronavirus that causes coronavirus disease 2019, or COVID-19)**

PROTOZOA

Cryptosporidium	cryptosporidiosis
Giardia lamblia	giardiasis
Plasmodium	malaria
Trypanosoma cruzi	chagas disease

FUNGI

Pneumocystis jiroveci pneumonia	opportunistic
Tinea	ringworm
Candida	candidiasis

PARASITES

Roundworm

Scabies

Tapeworm

Flatworm

PROTEINS

Prion   BSE, VCJD

Insert from Constance
From all that I have read and understood on this subject over the years, it seems that the purpose of pathogens is to decompose. If an organism dies, plant, or animal, it needs to decompose.

When the body's pH level is not balanced, mostly too acidic, the body sends a vibration out to the universe, a message that it is deteriorating. Thus, the universe responds by sending a message to the pathogens to come and do their job; decompose and clean up.

Medical reason of transmission of pathogens is through air, touch, food, or water becoming contaminated (physical body). The <u>holistic</u> reason for pathogens is simply this plus the person's mental, emotional, and spiritual state. Meaning that you attract energy to you depending on your own body's vibration.

Vibratory rate (hertz) is how fast the cells are moving. An example is when you think bad thoughts the vibratory rate of your cells changes. Scientists have medically proven that the chemistry of a teardrop from the eye changes due to the emotions being felt at the time; happy, sad, angry, etc.

The late Dr. Valerie Hunt had been doing extensive research in the field of vibratory healing. http://www.bioenergyfields.org/ and found that a person with let us say cancer, vibrates at about half of the average person's rate, and if you change the vibratory rate of the person, their condition in many cases will change.

There is also information on 'what you think changes the way food is processed in your body.'

An example that was given in an herb course I took had a diagram of a young lady sitting on a park bench on a beautiful afternoon. It looked like she was eating a healthy vegetarian lunch while a businessman is sitting beside her, eating a hamburger and fries. She is looking at him in disgust, and he is oblivious to her as he is enjoying his moment in the sun away from his hectic day. The meaning was to be careful of what you think.

Stress is the number one concern to a natural health or spa practitioner. *The lady's vibration at that moment was worse than the man's due to her thoughts.*

Infection – Immunity

What protection does our body have to infection?
- Mouth
- Stomach acid
- Skin
- Mucus
- Lymph
- T-cells
- Hair –body, eyelashes, nose & ears

What areas of our body do we need to be concerned with?
- Eyes
- Ears
- Nose
- Mouth
- Vaginal/Penis
- Anal
- Open cuts

How can we protect ourselves?
- Gloves
- Stay healthy
- Aromatherapy
- Clean hands
- Clean equipment
- Do not touch our own face

First Aid

If an emergency, call 911
Have on hand a first aid kit, tea tree, alum, and saline solution.

Bleeding
- Scratch someone with your nail
- Nose
- Menstruation
- Anal & Urinary (hydrotherapy)
- Dry brushing before a massage

Burns (anything that can cause immediate or after in the sun/tanning)
- Hot Rock Massage
- Pedi/Mani
- Hydrotherapy
- Aromatherapy product
- Heated blankets
- Thai herbal massage products

Choking
Fainting
Eye Injury

Sanitization Rules

What does a client care about?
- Dirt & dust
- Fluff on the floor
- Garbage cans
- Smells
- Clean equipment
- Clean laundry
- Your body odor – breath, underarms (female menstruation)
- Dirty nails
- The place is tidy & organized

Esthetics, Massage, or Nails *(under normal circumstances)*

Greet client

Seat client

The health form is filled out

Practitioner sanitizes their own hands with an antibacterial soap.

Session procedure - Use of tools:

- Metal
- Sanitisable
- Disposable

End of session

Clean up

- All disposable items are put into the garbage and disposed of each night.
- All station garbage is emptied before each new client arrives.
- Towels and sheets are put into the laundry hamper and washed during the day.
- All surfaces are cleaned and sprayed with bleach and/or rubbing alcohol.
- Metal tools are washed and then put into T36 disinfectant hospital grade for a minimum of 20 minutes.
- Sanitizable tools are washed and sprayed with rubbing alcohol
- Massage tables and headrests are washed and sprayed with rubbing alcohol. I, Connie, have never had a blood-stained massage table sheets in the last nine years, but if you did, you would just dispose of them, which would be put into a separate plastic bag and throw into the garbage. *Bleach???*
- Headrests are covered in protective cotton fabric or disposable, a new one with every client.
- Sheepskin covers on the massage tables are washed in the washing machine weekly or as needed.
- Floor mats are washed in the washing machine, weekly or as needed.
- Washrooms are lightly cleaned daily and scrubbed down three times in five days or more if needed.
- Floors are swept or vacuumed daily or as needed. Corners included furniture is moved once per week.
- Water coolers have disposable cups.
- All Staff must be in clean clothes daily and well-groomed.

- All products are put into separate disposable containers with each client. A disposable spoon is used to fill or is washed each time.
- No double-dipping into any product or wax.
- Glass or stainless-steel mixing containers are used. No plastic or wood.
- We do not use needles or any other sharp disposable items.
- All sponges are disposed of after each client unless they can be washed in a washing machine.
- All ventilation is checked yearly.
- Clarite Artificial nails non-smelling product is used. When filing, the nail's practitioner can use a mask.

Blood spill procedure:
- Stop the service and wash your hands.
- Cover your hands with protective gloves.
- Supply the injured party with a styptic powder or spray and the appropriate dressing to cover the injury.
- Do not allow containers, brushes, nozzles, or styptic containers to touch the skin or come into contact with the wound.
- Disinfect the station and implements with a disinfectant.
- Double bag all disposable, blood-soiled articles and discard, making sure that it is sealed to protect anyone from coming in contact with the material.

If the practitioner hurts themselves, they need to stop service and wash, disinfect, and cover with a bandage or wear plastic gloves.

Sanitization Products

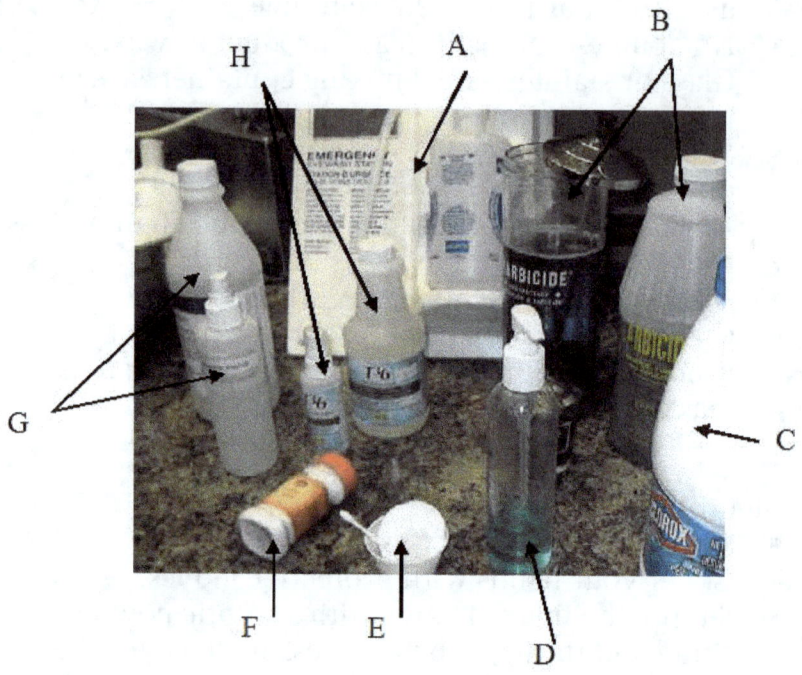

Items you will need if you have any type of Spa, Health or Beauty business.

- A. Saline Solution - to wash out eyes (Brow & Lash Tinting)
- B. Barbacide – great for plastic items
- C. Bleach – towels or blood spillage
- D. Hand sanitizer
- E. Disposable items
- F. Alum – blood issues on fingers or toes
- G. Rubbing Alcohol – spray to clean metal, tabletops, hot rocks or massage beds
- H. T36 – spray on metal items, kills even HIV

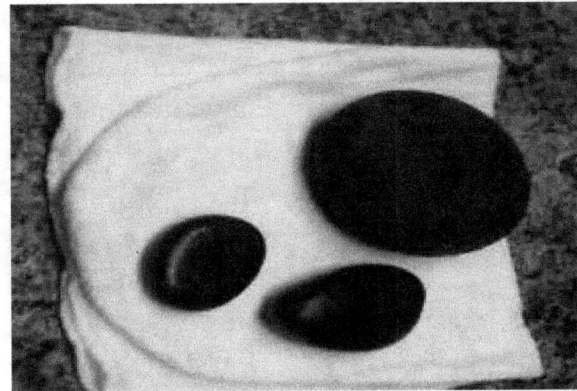

Hot Rocks: Wash with soap and water, then after they dry spray with rubbing alcohol.

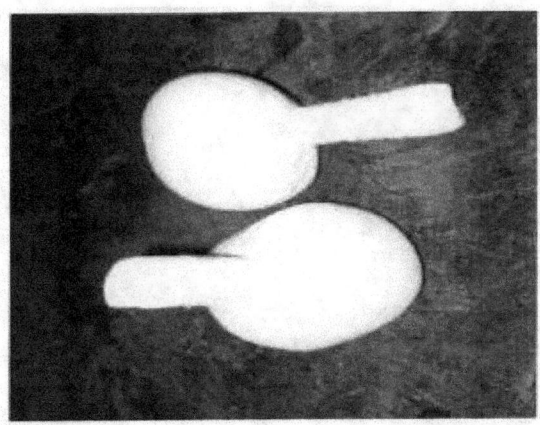

Items like these: Herbs for Thai Massage
Give it to the client or throw away. They cannot be cleaned after being used!

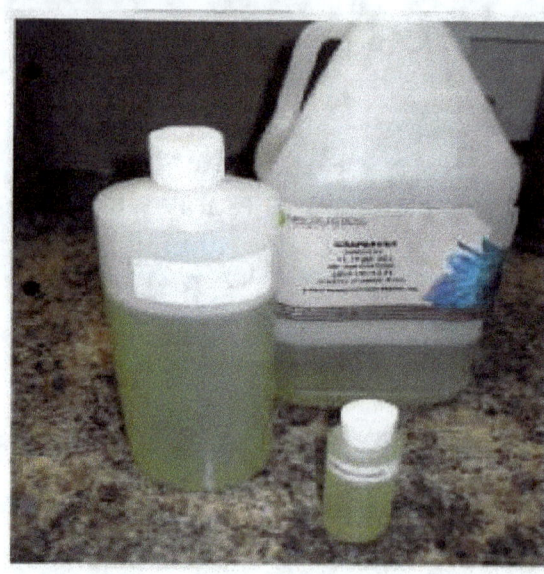

**When you have purchased a larger item and have put it into smaller containers, make sure you have LABLED the new containers.

Spa Techniques

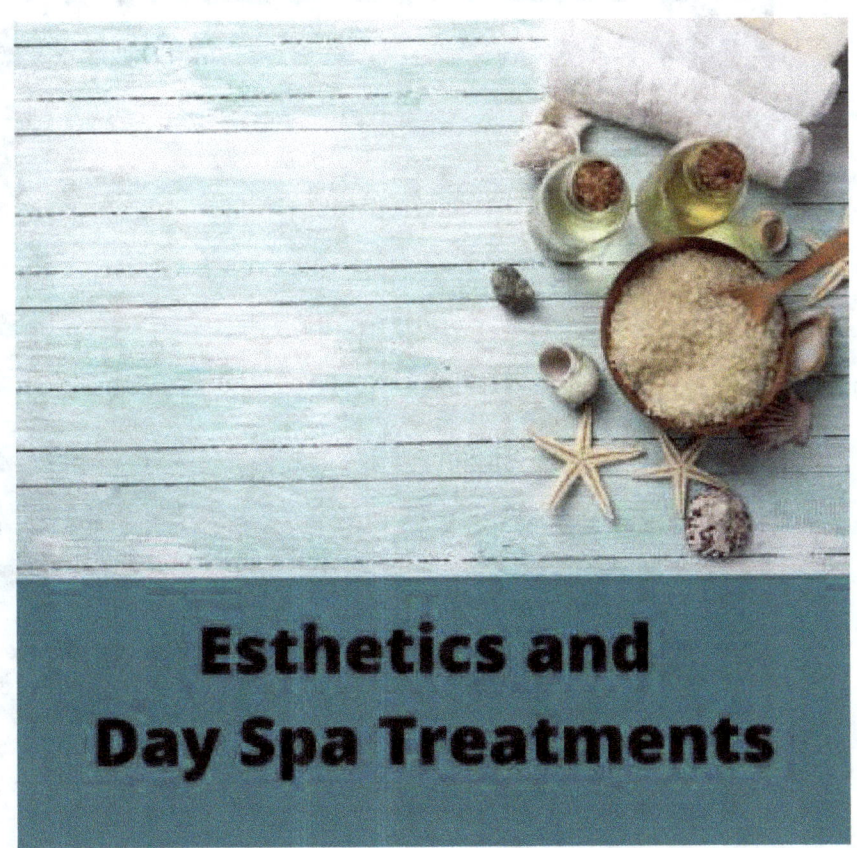

Esthetics and Day Spa Treatments

Mani's

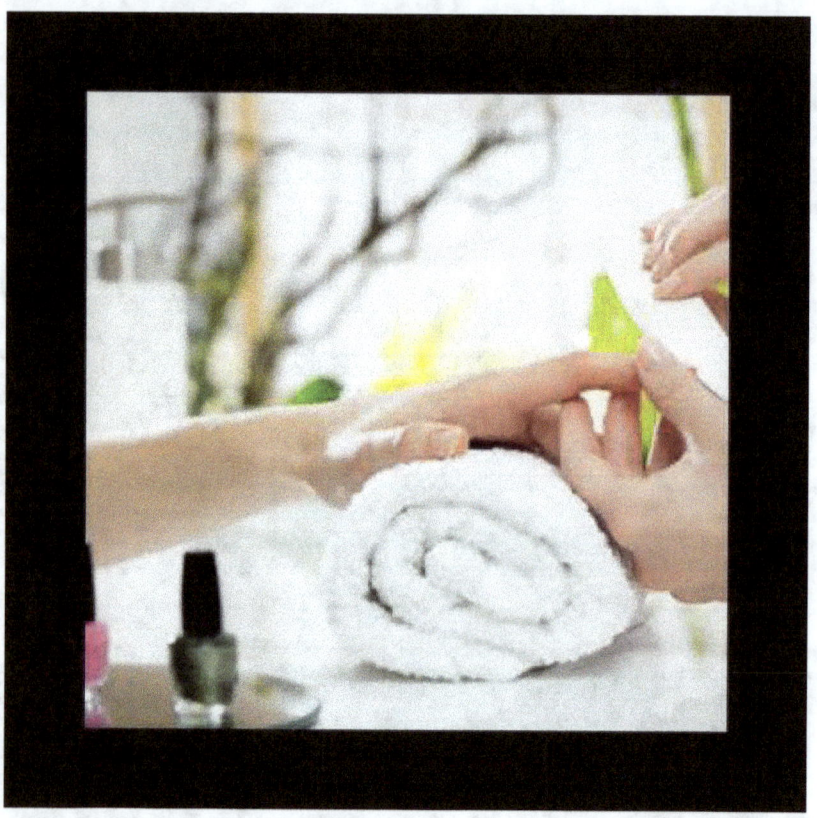

The difference between a Mani-care and Manicure.

Mani-care is the care of the nails, pampering them. (*No manipulation of the nail is allowed, other than filing*).

Manicure is where we can remove the cuticle and clip nails, and the use of metal tools.

History

The first manicures did not require any formal instruction. The word manicure comes from the Latin "manus" (hand) and "cura" (care). The evidence of nail care recorded in history was before 3000 BC in Egypt and China. Ancient Egyptian men and women of high social rank stained their nails with a red-orange dye called henna, which comes from a shrub. The color of a person's nails in ancient Egypt was a sign of importance. Kings and Queens wore deep red, white people of lower rank could wear only paler colors.

Around 3000 BC the Chinese developed nail paint made from beeswax, egg whites, gelatin, and gum Arable. In 600 BC Chinese royalty wore gold and silver paint on their nails for beauty and as well as stature. In the 15th century, leaders of the Chinese Ming dynasty painted their nails black and red. Military commanders in Egypt Babylon and early Rome spent hours before a battle having their hair lacquered and curled, and their nails painted the same shade as their lips.

PARTS OF THE NAIL:

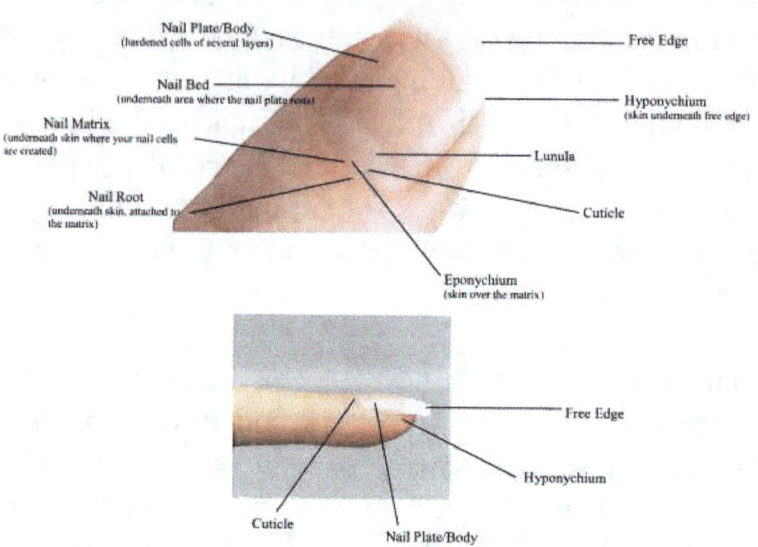

The actual nail consists of:

- nail body,
- nail root,
- free edge.

The nail body or plate is the main part or plate of the nail that is attached to the skin at the tip of the finger. Although the nail plate appears to be one piece, it is constructed of layers.

The nail root is where nail growth begins. It is embedded underneath the skin at the base of the nail.

The free edge is the end of the nail that extends beyond the fingertip.

STRUCTURES BENEATH THE NAIL:

The structure beneath the nail includes the nail bed, matrix, and lunula. The nail bed is the portion of the skin beneath the nail body that the nail plate rests upon. The nail bed is supplied with blood vessels that provide nourishment necessary for nail growth. The nail bed also consists of nerves.

The matrix contains nerves together with lymph and blood vessels that produce nail cells and control the rate of growth of the nail. It is located under the nail and, if injured, will produce nails with irregular growth disorders. The lunula is the light color half-moon shape at the base of the nail. This is where the matrix connects with the nail bed.

SKIN SURROUNDING THE NAIL:

The skin surrounding the nail includes the cuticle, nail fold, nail grooves, nail wall, eponychium, perionychium, and hyponychium.

- The cuticle if the overlapping skin around the nail. A normal cuticle should be loose and pliable.
- The nail fold or mantle is the deep fold of skin at the base of the nail where the nail root is embedded.
- The nail grooves are slits or tracks in the nail bed at the sides of the nail on which the nail grows.
- The nail wall is the skin on the sides of the nail above the grooves.
- The eponychium is the thin line of skin at the base of the nail that extends from the nail wall to the nail plate.

- The perionychium is the part of the skin that surrounds the entire nail area.
- The hyponychium is the part of the skin under the free edge of the nail.

Nails & Nail Diseases

Why, oh why, oh why are we learning this stuff, you may be asking yourself? The real reason is some of you are learning this for a profession, and you will be working with other professionals that may or may not know more than you. It is crucial that you know how to recognize these diseases so you can handle a situation if it arises.

This information may seem like common sense but for some, it can be difficult when placed in a situation to know what to say or even how to say it tactfully.

As a spa practitioner or esthetician, you will be doing many, many mani-cares or manicures, but not before you know what to look for and what to be careful of.

NAIL DISORDERS:

A nail disorder is a condition caused by injury to the nail or disease or imbalance in the body. Most clients will have at one time or another had one or another kind of nail imperfection or imbalance. They may even come to you with a disease to be treated by educating yourself on what you can do a service on and what you cannot, you protect yourself and your client from the spread of something that could be communicable.

THE GOLDEN RULE IS:

IF THE NAIL OR SKIN TO BE WORKED ON IS INFECTED, INFLAMED, BROKEN, OR SWOLLEN, YOU SHOULD NOT SERVICE THE CLIENT.

NAIL DISORDER THAT YOU <u>CAN</u> SERVICE:

Bruised nails; is a condition in which a clot of blood forms under the nail plate. The clot is usually caused by an injury to the nail bed.

Discolored nails: this is a condition in which the nails turn a variety of colors, including yellow, blue, grey, green, red & purple. Discoloration can be caused by poor blood circulation, a heart condition, or topical or oral medications.

Eggshell nails: are thin, white, and curved over the free edge. The condition is caused by improper diet, internal disease, medication, or nervous disorders.

Furrows: also known as corrugations, are long ridges that run either lengthwise or across the nail. Furrows are normal and increase with age.

Hangnails: also known as agnail is a common condition caused by the cuticle becoming dry and splitting. Keeping the cuticles moist and oil will help this condition greatly.

Leukonychia: is a condition in which white spots appear on the nail. It can be caused by injury and will usually grow out.

Onychophagy: Is bitten nails that have been bitten enough to become deformed. This condition can be greatly improved with regular use of manicare or manicures.

CANNOT BE SERVICED! Send to a Doctor

- Mold Fungus: Yellow / Green & darkens to Black. When Moisture seeps between natural nail & artificial nail.
- Onychia: Red, swollen, pus
- Onychoeryphosis: the curvature of the nail is increased & enlarged nail becomes thicker & curves results in inflammation and pain if it grows into the skin.
- Onychomycosis: (tinea uniguium) 1st whitish patches that can be scraped off. 2nd form long yellowish streaks. An infectious disease caused by a fungus (vegetable parasite).
- Onycholysis: Nail loosens from the nail bed, beginning at the free edge, continuing to lunula, but does not come off. Internal disorder, trauma, infection, or certain drug treatments hand or feet.
- Onychoptosis: Sheds & falls off. Occur during or after certain diseases such as syphilis, fever, and trauma or reaction to prescription drugs.

SPA MANI-CARE PROCEDURE

Items and products needed:

- Notes to perform manicure treatment *(in poly pockets while learning the procedure)*
- Four hand towels
- Box of tissues
- Gibson or tissue
- Hand sanitizer
- Damp cotton wool squares
- Cotton wool pads
- Nail enamel remover
- Emery boards
- Manicure bowl
- Hand soak
- Cuticle massages cream/oil
- Cuticle remover
- Exfoliant
- Mask and or paraffin wax
- Plastic liners and gloves
- Hindu stick or hoof stick
- Two orangewood sticks, lined at tips with cotton wool
- Paraffin wax brush
- Nail brush
- Massage medium, oil/cream
- Buffing paste
- Buffer
- Ridge filler (optional)
- Basecoat
- Nail enamel (various colors, including frosted and French manicure). Check varnish is of the right consistency and thin if necessary
- Topcoat

- 2 small bowls; one for client's jewelry (lined with tissue) and one for cotton wool
- Alcohol
- Waste bag or can
- Dappen dish for cuticle remover (tiny glass dish)
- Spatulas
- Large bowl for water
- Towels or sponges for removal of exfoliant

NAIL SUPPLIES AND PRODUCT INFO

Files/buffers:

Use disposable or sanitizable files only.

- Disposable files can be thrown away after each session or can be given to the client to take home. Never clean and use it on a second client!
- Sanitizable (cleanable) Scrub down with soap & water using a nail brush, then spray with rubbing alcohol. Let dry.

File types

100 grit – very coarse, used for very thick toenails

180 grit – medium-coarse, used for toenails

240 grit –fine coarse, used for fingernails and can be used as a buffer for toenails

3 color buffer (this has three different grits on one file)

Great for making the nails shiny.

Do not use if painting the nails with nail polish.

Toenails

- can be filed in both directions
- should be soaked in water to soften the nail
- plastic toe separators must be thrown away after each use. Can use folded Kleenex

Fingernails

- are very soft and can only be filed in one direction to avoid weakening the nail
- can be filed dry or wet (do not soak for very long)

Client's care most about the looks of the shape of the nail, free edge (under the nail), and cuticle. Ask your client their preference.

Orangewood stick is to be thrown away after each use.

Products:

- **Cleaner-** used to soak finger or toes in
- **Cuticle remover-** for thick cuticles will dissolve the skin
- **Oil** – used to soften and treat dry skin
- **Peel/exfoliate-** used to remove dead skin cells
- **Paraffin dip** (do not have to do) – used with cream to promote soft skin
- **Cream or oil-** to massage in and leave arms and hands soft
- **Nail polish-**
    - Basecoat - to protect the nail bed
    - Polish – to color the nail (use two coats)
    - Topcoat – to prevent chipping
    - Quick-dry sprays - to help speed up drying time

SPA MANI-CARE PROCEDURE

1. Prepare all products, instruments, towels, etc. *It is important to be fully prepared before your client arrives.*
2. Wash and sanitize your hands
3. Sanitize workstation
4. Remove all jewelry
5. Lay towel no.1 on the table vertically
6. Roll towel no.2 in the center of your work area
7. Lay Gibson or tissue on top of the rolled towel
8. Fold towel no.3 and place at the side of the work area
9. Set out the remaining items on the trolley in the order that you will use them
10. Cover remaining items with a small towel
11. Towel no.4 is placed on the practitioner's knee to protect clothing.
12. Some clients like to pay ahead, so they do not scratch their new nail polish
13. Greet your client, then seat her/him comfortably.
14. Fill out client consultation; place all notes on the lower shelf of the trolley.
15. If client is a new customer, briefly explain the procedure.

Treatment should take approximately 45 minutes.

Client care

1. Wash and sanitize your hands and the clients.
2. There are different thought patterns regarding which hand the practitioner should start with. The working hand is normally soaked for longer.

Canadian associations normally prefer the left hand).
3. Ask your client to choose a nail color.
4. Fill manicure bowl with warm water and add hand soak.
5. Ask client to roll up their sleeves and remove their jewelry, place jewelry in tissue-lined small bowl.
6. **Check for contra-indications**, then add to notes if necessary.
7. Remove old polish from both hands with cotton pads; **check all nails for contra-indications.**

Filing

8. File and shape the nails on the working hand using an emery board, asking the client which shape they prefer. Bevel the nail to avoid the nail layers splitting apart. Use the emery board at a **45-degree angle** to the nail and file **one way only**, from the side to the center. Do not saw the nail. This causes peeling due to the heat effect. Do not file the corners of the nail.
9. Apply and massage a cuticle cream/oil onto the cuticles, then place the client's hand in the manicure bowl, covering with a small towel to keep hand warm.
10. **Repeat 7 and 8 on the other hand.**

- *The quality of the job you do on the foundation (nail prep) will determine the end result once the nail polish is on.*
- *File in one direction only. The fingernail is thin, and back and forth will weaken the nail.*
- *When filing, make sure not to file into the corner of the nails as this will make the nail weak.*

- *If you file the nails dry, you will have more control of the shape.*
- *Most practitioners start from a pinky finger and work their way through both hands. Habit is to work so that your hand is not going to drag across wet nail polish.*

Nail Shapes

Many people like a different shape when you file their nails.

Choices:

- Oval nails
- Pointed nails
- Rectangular or Square nails *(most popular today)*
- Round nails
- Flat corners

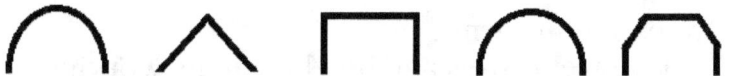

Cuticle work

11. Lift hand from manicure bowl and pat dry.
12. Scrub nails with brush
13. Clean under free edge using orangewood stick.
14. Dry the hand.
15. Dip Hindu stick in cuticle remover and gently push the cuticles back.
16. Remove dead skin cells from nail plate with a Hindu stick. Using small circular movements, keeping stick wet at all times.
17. Repeat on the other hand.

18. Oil cuticles on both hands, starting with the pinky finger.
19. Remove the manicure bowl

Science is saying that a cuticle should be there to help prevent disease.

- Need to be soaked to be able to push back and shape
- A wet Hindu stick / Pumice stone can be used to help remove dead skin
- Wet cotton wrapped orangewood stick can be used to clean or shape the cuticle

Exfoliation

Need two warm wet towels (wring out water).

20. Exfoliate right and left hand and arm, using light effleurage movements and remove with sponges or towels.
21. Dry hands and arms.
22. Remove wet towels and bowl from the working area.

Mask treatment

23. **Optional** – apply paraffin wax to hand and wrist area (This is a good time to tidy up the trolley or talk to the client about hand and nail care, home care, etc., while the wax is cooling.)

Massage

24. Protect clients clothing

25. Apply massage cream evenly onto the client's hand and arm and perform a massage.

HAND AND ARM MASSAGE

- Protect clients' clothing at the elbow with a tissue.
- Take massage medium and warm in palms of your hands.
- Spread medium evenly from fingertips to elbow.
- Check to make sure the client's hand and arm is comfortable on towel roll and ask her to relax arm and hand.
- Place your hand in a 'shake hands' position with the clients.
- Effleurage from fingertips to elbow, finger circling at elbow x 5
- Turn the client's hand over and 'link your thumb with the clients.
- Effleurage from the fingertips to the elbow crease x 5.
- Thumb circles to carpals x 5
- Thumb strokes in between metacarpals x 5
- Knead thumb and palm pad x 5.
- Finger kneading from fingertips to finger base, slide down to the second phalange, support joint and turn finger clockwise and anti-clockwise x 3. Slide off finger using a vibration movement.
- Bend client's arm and thumb knead palm of hand x 5.
- Clasp your hand around the client's wrist above carpals and turn wrist clockwise and anti-clockwise with other hand x 3.
- Thumb knead clients palm x 5

- Finger tap front and back of the arm (Tapotement) x 5
- Effleurage

26. Remove excess massage cream if necessary.
27. *Squeak,* using nail polish remover, the nails to remove any excess cream or lotion.

Buffing *(if not using nail polish)*

28. Apply oil to each nail (which should be the size of a pinhead) using an orangewood stick.
29. Buff nails; going in the direction of the nail growth.
30. Ask the client to put their jewelry back on.

Nail Polish

31. Ask the client to choose nail color.
32. Apply **basecoat,** *(practice using three strokes: center and each side)* to all ten nails, starting with the little finger on the left hand. *Trying not to flood cuticle.*
33. Apply **two coats** of nail enamel (nail polish), using **three strokes**
34. Let dry
35. Apply a **topcoat**, using **three strokes**.
36. **Wash and sanitize your hands**
37. **Complete client card** and give client **aftercare** advice: *(see aftercare advice notes).* Record the color of nail enamel chosen by the client, the next appointment time, update any other information, and add any other comments that are relevant to the treatment. **Make sure the client has all her/his belongings before leaving the area.**
38. Take the **client to reception** to pay and make another appointment if she so desires.

39. **Wash and sanitize** all the tools and throw away used disposables, and clean and sanitize the work area before leaving room.
40. **Wash and sanitize your hands** before leaving the treatment room.

AFTERCARE ADVICE FOR MANI

1. Wear gloves when doing household chores/gardening
2. Do not use the nails as tools
3. Apply cuticle oil every evening
4. Apply hand cream at least twice a day
5. Use the correct technique when filing, do not saw
6. Always use basecoat before applying nail polish
7. Advise the client on a treatment plan to improve their nail and skin conditions, and the time intervals between each treatment
8. Advise on appropriate nail/skincare products to remedy any problems
9. Keep an emery board in their purse to use on ragged edges
10. Do not pull or bite the skin around the nails
11. Do not file into the corners of nails
12. Exfoliate hands regularly

*Your client may like to talk to you with this service, and it is nice to get to know her or him. Find out what they do etc. Remember, this is your client's session, not yours. Listen!

Note: It may take several sessions to create beautiful nails. A client who works hard with their hands may take 3 -5 sessions.

QUICK **MANI-CARE** PROCEDURE

Start on their Left hand, pinky finger.
1. Examine their nails.
2. **File** and shape nails (file in one direction only) 240 grit file. Continue onto the right hand.
3. Excuse yourself and fill the mani bowl with warm water (put **cleanser product** in the bowl, -citrus soak and/or sea fizz or another brand) and ask your client to begin soaking their right hand
4. **Clean cuticles** using orange stick wrapped in a bit of cotton and Hindu / pumice stone, using the other end of the orange stick for under the nail. Continue onto the right hand.
5. **Oil** (e.g. grapeseed, jojoba, almond, or olive) rub into cuticles of one hand starting with the pinkie finger. Continue onto right hand.
6. Massage in **exfoliant** from elbow to fingertips and remove with warm hot towels (this is a 2-step procedure with some product lines). Continue onto the right hand.
7. Optional! Apply ample cream on hands then do a **Paraffin dip.** Let sit 5-20 min. in plastic covers, and then remove all of the wax.
8. Do **massage.** Apply cream or oil on one arm at a time.
9. To prepare the surface for painting, clean oil/lotions off nails with nail polish remover. **Paint nails** (1 coat of base, 2 coats of color, 1 coat of topcoat). Remove any extra polish off the skin once the polish has dried. If not painting the nails, buff with a three-surface buffing file.

Tools

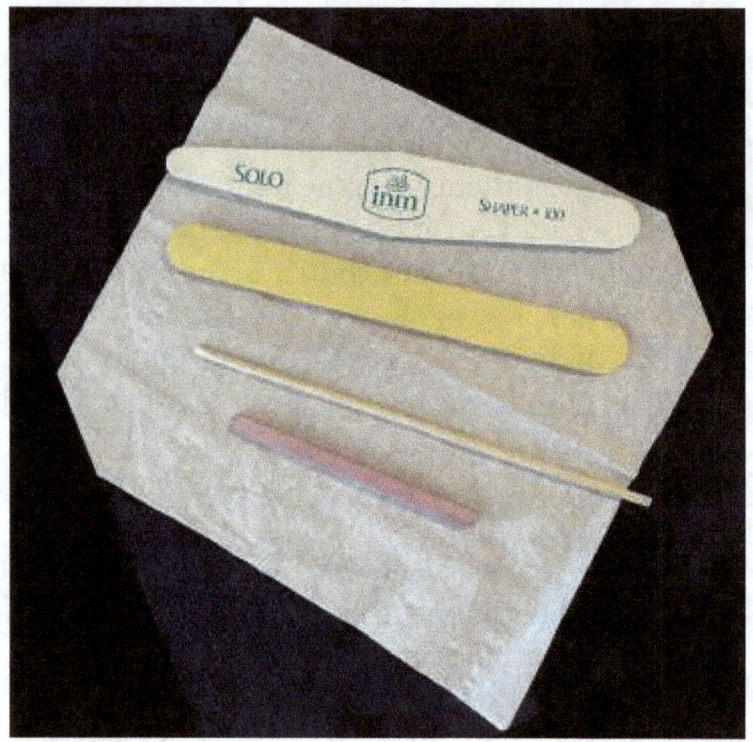

Files 100/180
Orangewood Stick
Hindu Stick/Pumice Stone

QUICK **MANICURE** PROCEDURE

Start on their Left hand, pinky finger.

1. Examine nails.
2. **File** and shape nails (file in one direction only) 240 grit file. Continue onto the right hand.
3. Excuse yourself and fill your mani bowl with warm water (put **cleanser product** in the bowl, -citrus soak and/or sea fizz or another brand) and ask your client to begin soaking their right hand
4. **Clean cuticles** using orange stick wrapped in a bit of cotton and Hindu / pumice stone, using the other end of the orange stick for under the nail. Continue onto the right hand.
5. **Nip cuticles** (hangnails or ragged cuticles)
6. **Oil** (e.g. grapeseed, jojoba, almond, or olive) rub into cuticles of one hand starting with the pinkie finger. Continue onto the right hand.
7. Massage in **exfoliant** from elbow to fingertips and remove with warm hot towels (this is a 2-step procedure with some product lines). Continue onto the right hand.
8. Optional! Apply ample cream on hands then do **Paraffin dip.** Let sit 5-20 min. in plastic covers, and then remove all of the wax.
9. Do **massage.** Apply cream or oil on one arm at a time.
10. To prepare the surface for painting, clean the oil/lotion off the nails with nail polish remover. **Paint nails** (1 coat of base, 2 coats of color, 1 coat of topcoat). Remove any extra polish off the skin once the polish has dried. If not painting the nails, buff with the three-surface buffing file.

Tools

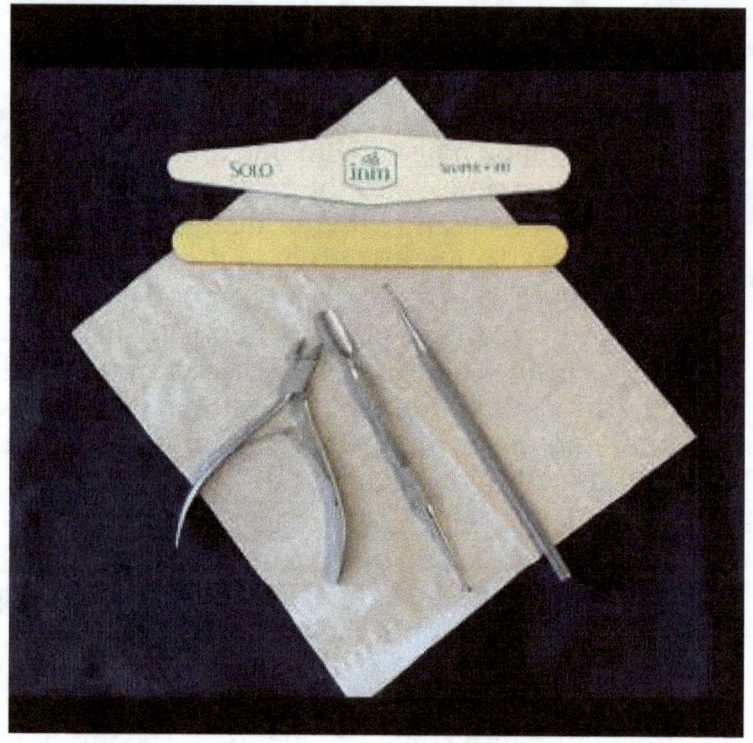

Files 100/180
Cuticle Nipper Long Handle Double Spring *(the blade can have different sizes, you may like using one more than another)*
Cuticle & Nail Pusher
Single Ended Excavator

BONUS: HOT OIL MANICURE

SUPPLIES:
Disposable Plastic Cups
Oils for the Heater
Refer to the Water Manicure Supply List
Hot Oil Heater

Items you may omit from the water manicure supply list are **Massage Lotion, Cuticle Solvent, and a Manicure Bowl.**

STATION SET UP:

- Refer to the Mani-care information.

PROCEDURE:

- Heat enough oil to cover the cuticles prior to the service.
- Have the client wash their hands with an antibacterial soap.
- Remove any polish.
- Shape the nails on the left hand.
- Remove any pterygium with a pumice stone.
- Place the left hand in the oil for 2-3 minutes.
- Shape the nails on the right hand.
- Remove any pterygium with a pumice stone.
- Place the right hand in the oil.
- With the left hand...
- Employ the soft cuticle pusher.
- Nip where necessary. (Checking for hangnails)

- Clean under the free edge.
- At this point, double check your work.
- Repeat these steps on the right hand.
- Using the oil from the heater, complete the manicure with the hand and arm massage.
- Remove any oil from the nail plate with a nail wipe and alcohol.
- Remove the excess oil from the client's arms using a warm towel, followed by a dry towel. (ensure that all the oil is off the client's hands and arms as it may stain their clothing)
- At this point, have your client take out their keys and put back on any jewelry they had worn.
- Apply the base coat.
- Apply the polish.
- Apply the topcoat.

Pedi's

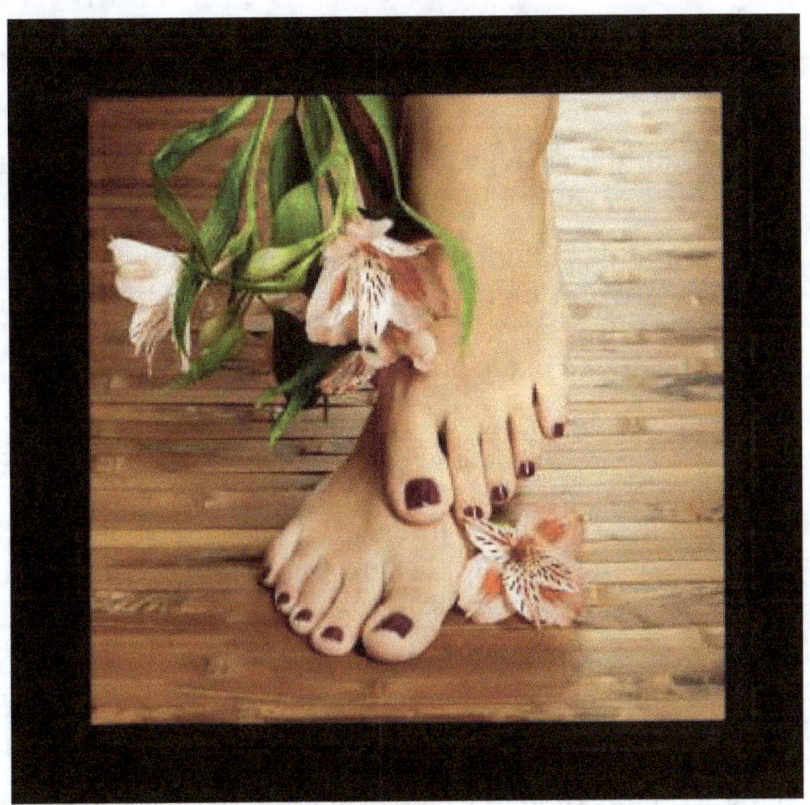

Foot Care

- Pedi-care
- Pedicurist
- Derma care nail specialists
- Foot Hygienist
- Nursing foot care Practitioner
- Podologist
- Podiatrist

Foot Care Practitioners can examine feet and toenails, trim nails by filing (estheticians and derma care nail specialists by also cutting), soak, exfoliate, apply paraffin mask, reduce the appearance of calluses using an emollient product, massage feet and lower-leg, and apply nail polish.

> **Cannot** use a lancet, gouge blade or other cutting blades, cannot diagnose or prescribe medication.

Foot Hygienists (Podologist) can treat foot discomfort and pain, prevent ingrown toenails, corns, calluses, etc., treat foot skin and nails, suggest creams, allowed to use lancet and gouge blade and assist podiatrist.

> **Cannot** diagnose or treat infections and wounds.

Foot Care Nurse can alleviate pain, prevent ingrown toenails, corns, calluses, fungus infections, etc., treat disease, wounds, and infections, prescribe over the counter creams and medications, educate.

Podiatrists can diagnose and treat foot disorders and disease using medical, chemical, pharmaceutical, and surgical, mechanical (braces) methods, or manipulations.

Many women come in to have a pedicure or pedi-care for esthetics, to look pretty. It is your responsibility to educate the client when they have a foot issue or disease (you cannot diagnose, but you can suggest that they go to a doctor or suggest products such as Footlogix and such).

Foot issues and diseases are on the rise, not because of conditions but due to age.

Since 2006, 25% of business in a Spa was Pedicures, with a 30% growth. As the baby boomers age, foot care is more and more in demand. Clients cannot bend as they did when younger; their circulation is not what it used to be either. This is a problem for the client when they cannot trim their own toenails or clean their own feet. The nail length can rub on other toes causing cuts and infection, be squeezed into shoes and cause pain and discomfort, become an area for pathogens and have ability to form major health issues.

Both, Men and women are coming in to have foot hygiene. We have a role in preventing problems, alleviating discomfort, and pain. It is the practitioner's job to clean and file the nails to an appropriate length (don't forget the love...and pamper...pamper...pamper).

Nail Supplies and Product Needed (similar to a mani):

Files/buffers:

Use disposable or sanitizable files only.

- Disposable files can be thrown away after each session or given to the client to take home. Never clean and use it on a second client!
- Sanitizable (cleanable) Scrub down with soap & water using a nail brush, then spray with rubbing alcohol. Let dry.

File types

100 grit – very coarse, used for very thick toenails

180 grit – medium-coarse, used for toenails

240 grit –fine coarse, used for fingernails and can be used as a buffer for toenails

3 color buffer (this has three different grits on one file)

Great for making the nails shiny.

Do not use if painting the nails with nail polish

Fort Toenails

- can be filed in both directions
- should be soaked in water to soften the nail
- plastic toe separators must be thrown away after each use. Can use folded Kleenex

For Fingernails

- are incredibly soft and can only be filed in one direction to avoid weakening the nail
- can be filed dry or wet (not soaked for very long)

Client's care most about the looks of the shape of nail, free edge (under the nail), and cuticle. Ask your client their preference.

*An orangewood stick is to be thrown away after each use.

Products:

- **Cleaner-** used to soak finger or toes in
- **Cuticle remover-** for thick cuticles will dissolve the skin
- **Oil –** used to soften and treat dry skin
- **Peel/exfoliant-** used to remove dead skin cells
- **Paraffin dip** (do not have to do) – used with cream to promote soft skin
- **Cream or oil-** to massage in and leave arms and hands soft
- **Nail polish-**
    - Base oat -to protect the nail bed
    - Polish – to color the nail (use two coats)
    - Topcoat – to prevent chipping
    - Quick-dry sprays- to help speed up drying time

Spa **Pedi-care** Procedure

Client care

- Make sure you have told the client to bring with them a pair of open-toed shoes!!!
- Prepare all products, foot baths, towels, etc. It is important to be fully prepared before your client arrives.
- Greet your client then get her seated.
- Do client consultation.
- Ask her to remove her shoes and any foot jewelry while you get her warm hot water. If you are using a foot bath that heats the water, you can have the water already.

Hygiene

1. **Sanitize your hands.** If having the client's foot on your lap, have a large towel placed across your lap.
2. Put both client's feet into the warm water 2-3 minutes. The client can pick out a nail polish color.
    Footbath - in warm water, add antibacterial soap (*sea rock soak crystals*). If using a vibrating foot bath, add a few drops of *foaming sea soak* also.
3. Dry and remove the feet one at a time and **examine the feet**.
4. Put the feet back into the water.
5. Remove foot from water & towel dry.

Prepare nail

6. **Remove nail polish.**

Cuticle

7. **Apply cuticle remover**
8. Use orangewood stick or Hindu stick (pumice stone) to **remove and push back cuticles** (sides only, not on the eponychium).
9. Use orangewood stick with no cotton and **clean under the free edge**.
10. Wash foot
11. Repeat on other foot
12. Apply **oil** onto the eponychium – massage into each nail.
13. Repeat on other foot
14. **Exfoliate** using *sea salt glow and/or peppermint*
15. Rinse & dry
16. Repeat on other foot

File

17. **Buff nail** - 240 grit (in the <u>direction</u> of the nail growth).
18. **File nail** the free edge of all the toes.

Skin surface

19. Apply *sea salt scrub* on dry on the leg all the way down to the foot and massage in and leave on for 2-3 minutes in the footbath.
20. Remove with a wet towel the scrub on the leg and foot.

21. If needed, apply a second *sea scrub*, apply to the leg all the way down the foot, and massage in. Leave on for 2-3 minutes in the footbath.
22. If needed, apply *sea serum* to calluses or dry spots (rinse your hands off after applying).
23. Dry off the foot. Wet the **Pedi paddle** then use on any callus area on the heel of the foot
24. Repeat on other foot
25. Remove foot from water, towel dry <u>foot,</u> and apply the *marine* **mask**.
26. Wrap foot (let stand for 2-5 min).
27. Repeat on other foot
28. Remove by putting foot & towel into water and then removing mask).
29. Dry both feet (do not put back into the water)
30. Optional - Apply lotion on foot and do Paraffin dip - let sit for 5-20 minutes. You can clean up your station while waiting.
31. Remove all wax.

Massage

32. First foot/leg and apply *massage oil or massage silk* – do a short foot & calf **massage.**

    -Effleurage -calf & foot (long strokes)

    -Petrissage -calf & foot (kneading with two hands up- 1 hand each side)

    -Friction calf (circular motion)

    -Massage heel (squeeze 6x)

    -Snowplow movement

    -Butterfly move

    -Toes (start at big toe – base to tip-pivot wrist)

-Friction foot (back & forth movement)

33. Repeat on other foot/leg
34. On extremely dry areas, apply a tiny amount of *cucumber heel therapy.*

Nail Polish

35. **Clean** any remaining oil or cream from **nails** with nail polish remover.
36. Clean **cuticles** a second time if needed
37. Buff with 1200 grit or **Apply the nail polish** to nails *(you might want to put the client's open-toed shoes on before applying the nail polish)* -1 base coat, 2 color coats, and 1 top coat to give the maximum length for the polish. (Toe separators are very handy, not cleanable). Your client may bring her favorite color.

* Remember to or have your secretary ask them about polish when they book an appointment and to bring open-toed shoes.

If the client did not bring open-toed shoes, tell the client to wait at least 20 minutes for the polish to dry. Nail polish will take overnight to harden.

If she is booked for more services with you, clean up while she is drying and prepare your next set-up for the next service. Keep checking on her and her polish. When her toes are dry to the touch (if you didn't put on her shoes before the nail polish), get her to slip on her sandals and walk with her to the door and see her off!

QUICK **PEDI-CARE** PROCEDURE

1. Complete form – get signed
2. Look at feet – contra-indications
3. Soak feet (stainless steel bowl)
4. File nails (buff only if not painting nails)
5. Clean under nails
6. Exfoliate feet & legs
7. Clean off
8. Pedi paddle bottom of feet
9. Clean off

Optional - Mask bottom of feet & clean off (remove foot bath)

Optional - Lotion for paraffin

10. Massage feet & legs
11. Clean nail bed with nail polish remover
12. Paint nails – 1 basecoat, 2 of the color, 1 topcoat

QUICK **PEDICURE** PROCEDURE

1. Complete form – get signed
2. Look at feet – contra-indications
3. Soak feet (stainless steel bowl)
4. File nails (buff only if not painting nails)
5. Clean under nails
6. *Nip cuticles (hangnails or ragged cuticles), it is suggested today, NOT to nip cuticles. They are there to protect the nail from damage and disease.
7. Exfoliate feet & legs
8. Clean off
9. Pedi paddle bottom of feet
10. Clean off

Optional - Mask bottom of feet & clean off (remove foot bath)

Optional - Lotion for paraffin

11. Massage feet & legs
12. Clean nail bed with nail polish remover
13. Paint nails – 1 basecoat, 2 of the color, 1 topcoat

Tools

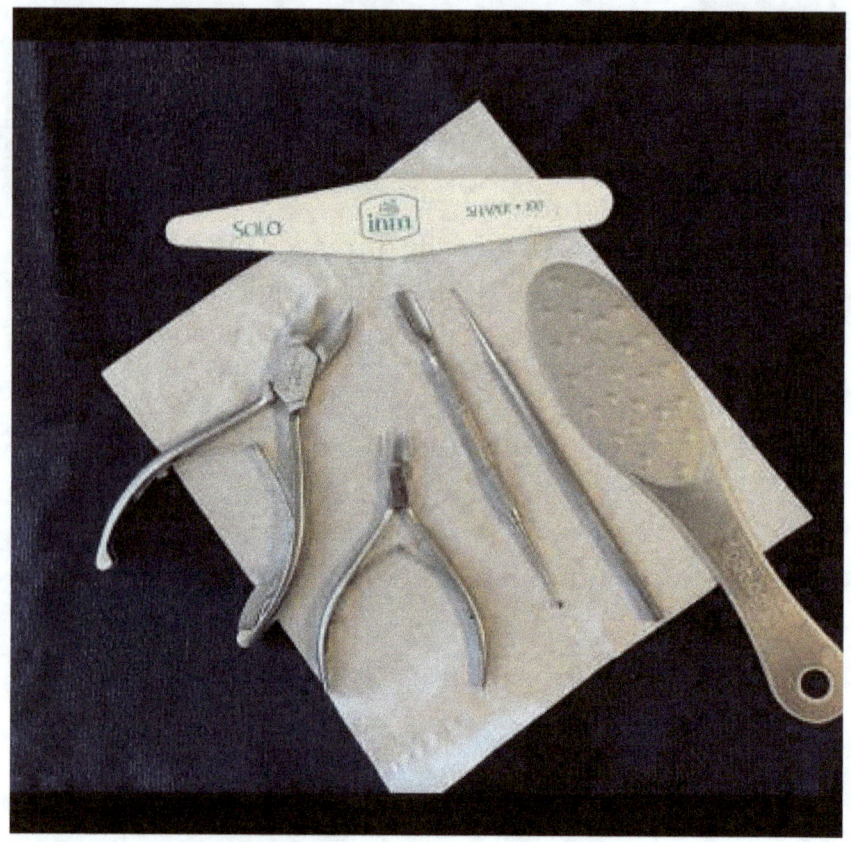

Files 80/100/180
Toenail Nipper Concave Jaw Double Spring
Pedicure & Ingrown Nail Nippers
Cuticle & Nail Pusher
Single Ended Excavator
Pedi paddle

Facials

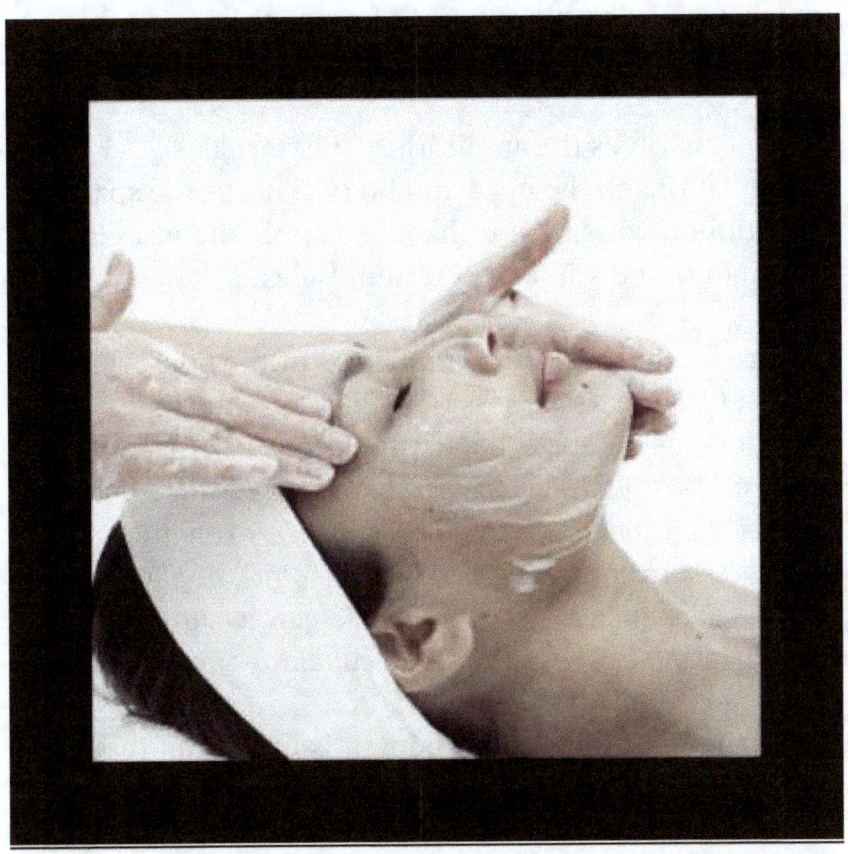

Benefits of Facial Massage

Let us talk a bit about why we incorporate massage with our facials. Facial massage is used to exercise the muscles in the face, maintain muscle tone, and stimulate circulation. As a spa practitioner, you will give massages to your clients to help keep their skin fresh and muscles firm.

To master the massage techniques, a spa practitioner must-have anatomy and physiology knowledge and, of course a considerable amount of practice in using the methods.

Massage involves the application of external manipulations to the head and body. You, as the spa practitioner, will use your hands to apply the massage movements and stimulate facial muscles.

You are limited to only certain areas of the body when doing a facial massage session: scalp, face, neck, shoulders, décolletage, hands, and arms.
Caution: *Do not give a massage without a doctor's note, when certain conditions exist, such as heart condition, high blood pressure, inflamed skin, swollen joints, or glandular swelling. Nor should you give a massage when abrasions of the skin, skin disorders, or broken capillaries are evident.*

To inspire confidence in a client, it is important that you give the massage with a firm, sure touch. To do this, you must develop strong, flexible hands, a quiet temperament, self-control, and the use of psychology. By having a thorough understanding of the facial muscles and nerves, you will be able to skillfully massage the right motor points, which will induce relaxation at the beginning of the session.

Facial massage will directly influence the structure and functions of the body. The Immediate effects of massage are first noticed on the skin. The section being massaged will respond by increased circulation, excretion, nutrition, and secretion.

The following beneficial results may be obtained by proper facial and scalp massage:

1. The skin and all its structures are nourished.
2. Fat cells in the subcutaneous tissue are reduced.
3. The skin is rendered soft and pliable.
4. The circulation of blood is increased.
5. The activity of the skin glands is stimulated.
6. The muscle fiber is stimulated and strengthened.
7. The nerves are soothed and rested.
8. Pain is sometimes relieved.

By keeping *your* hands soft (by using creams, oils, and lotions), you will make sure your client receives the most comfortable massage. Beveling your nails and keeping them smooth will reduces the possibility of accidentally scratching your client. The use of creams, oils, and ointments will also reduce the friction and drag on your clients' tender skin.

Not only do you use these movements in facial massage, but you also use them in other areas as well and in full body massage. Get to know these movements and their names. It is important to realize that with good technique and some practice and your extensive knowledge of anatomy that these massage movements contribute to a very positive experience for your client. Your client will get to realize and see the difference over time that the facials with massage can make. This helps you to establish a good relationship with your client when they can see that you are making a difference and not only just performing a service.

By using your knowledge and by establishing a fluent routine in all aspects of massage, you will increase your income as well. More clients will book appointments with you as word of mouth spreads about your services, and the way you perform them as well.

Practicing with your family and friends will also help you build confidence in your service and your clients will feel your reassuring touch when they come to you for treatments. As a Spa Practitioner, you want to reassure them with your touch in all aspects of your treatments. I would encourage you to practice as much as possible.

SKIN TYPES

Normal
Normal skin is soft, smooth, supple & not prone to eruptions. Healthy glow.

Dry
Dry skin is characterized by coarse and poreless appearance with fine lines, especially around the eyes and mouth. Dry skin lacks moisture because of under functioning sebaceous glands.

Oily
Oily skin tends to develop blackheads, whiteheads, and enlarged pores. An oily skin condition is caused by over-functioning sebaceous glands. Because pores can be clogged with make-up and debris as well as oil.
Shiny, sallow (yellowy, pasty), and often has open pores, black heads, and acne.

Combination
Combination skin is characterized by a poreless and smooth appearance on the cheeks, but with enlarged, clogged pores on the nose, forehead, and chin.
Oily section — usually forehead, nose, chin, and areas of dry skin

Problem
Problem/oily skin is characterized by an oily and shiny appearance with a tendency to develop blackheads, whiteheads, and pimples. Surface dryness may also be experienced due to improper cleansing with alkaline soap

or harsh acetone-based astringents. Prone to blackheads, acne &spots. Often oily.

Sensitive
Sensitive skin reacts readily to various factors such as specific chemicals, airborne debris, or certain skincare ingredients (fragrance and chemical preservatives top the list). Symptoms of sensitive skin include blotchiness, breakouts, or excessive dryness. Dry, prone to flaking, itching, redness, a tendency to allergic reactions, and broken capillaries.

Mature
Mature skin loses elasticity and its ability to retain moisture. With signs of aging - fine lines, wrinkles, and sagging.

Facial Needs

Normal skin

It is soft, smooth, supple, and not prone to eruptions and has a healthy glow.

    Cleanser:
- Cleansing
- Moisturizing

    Toner:
- Removing surface impurities.
- Hydrating
- Tone and balance the pH of the skin

    Scrub:
- Cleans pores & remove impurities
- Hydrate

    Masque:
- Detoxifying

    Serum:
- rejuvenate

    Moisturizer:
- Hydrating
- Antioxidant

Oily skin

It is shiny, sallow (yellow & pasty), often has open pores, black heads, and acne.

Cleanser:

- Deep cleansing

Toner:

- Mattifying and normalizing
- Hydrating and soothing

Scrub:

- Cleans pores & remove impurities
- Honey to hydrate
- Zinc oxide to calm skin & help heal

Masque:

- detoxify and clarify acne
- anti-blemish
- minimizing enlarged pores

Serum:

- Treats blemishes, spots and acne, control shine, reduce redness, irritation, and hormonally imbalanced skin types.

Moisturizer:

- Light moisturizer to regulate oily, over-reactive skin

Combination skin

It has oily sections (usually the forehead, nose, and chin) and areas of dryness.

Cleanser:

- Cleansing
- Acne control
- Moisturizing

Toner:

- Removing surface impurities.
- Hydrating
- Tone and balance the pH of the skin

Scrub:

- Cleans pores & remove impurities
- Hydrate
- Calm skin & help heal

Masque:

- Anti-blemish
- Detoxifying

Serum:

- Treat blemishes,
- Irritation
- Hormonally imbalanced skin

Moisturizer:

- Hydrating
- Antioxidant

Problem skin

Is prone to blackheads, acne, spots, and is often oily, may have Rosacea.

Cleanser:

- Deep cleansing

Toner:

- Mattifying and normalizing
- Hydrating and soothing

Scrub:

- Cleans pores & remove impurities
- Honey to hydrate
- Zinc oxide to calm skin & help heal

Masque:

- detoxify and clarify acne
- anti-blemish
- minimizing enlarged pores

Serum:

- Treats blemishes, spots and acne, control shine, reduce redness, irritation, and hormonally imbalanced skin types.

Moisturizer:

- Light moisturizer to regulate oily, over-reactive skin

Sensitive Skin

It is dry and prone to flaking, itchy, redness, tendency to allergic reactions, and broken capillaries.

Cleanser:
- Hydrating & lightweight (moisturizes)
- Not oily, drying or heavy (thus not clogging pores)

Toner:
- Calms the sensitive skin
- Reduces irritation to treat the sensitivity
- Tones the skin while removing surface impurities.

Scrub:
- Cleans pores & remove impurities
- High quantities of Vit 'C' (antioxidants)
- Honey to hydrate
- Zinc oxide to calm skin & help heal

Masque:
- Healing benefits.
- Irritation is reduced & complexion is healed.
- Soothing & nourishing
- Help to prevent breakouts.

Serum:
- Couperose 'C' serum
- Anti-irritant & antioxidant
- Reduces inflammation & irritation
- Calming & antiseptic
- Skin's immunity against free radicals
- Helps halt & stabilize visible signs of rosacea

Moisturizer:

- Lightweight
- Not greasy
- Reduce sebum production
- Discourage unwanted blemishes
- Corrective moisturizer

***

*At the Vancouver Esthétique Spa International Conference and Trade Show, the man who usually is there displaying his 'Eminence Organic Skin Care' line, is a hoot! If you get a chance to see one of his classes, go, it is worth waiting for.

This conference is a must for Spa and Esthetic students and spa owners. Sorry, it is not open to the public.

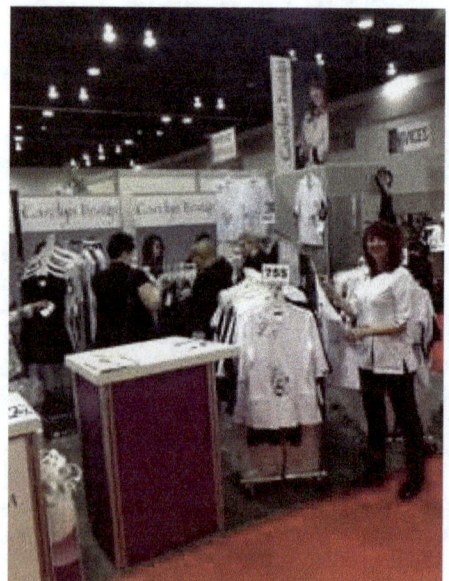

Check out Carolyn Designs while you are there, she offers beautiful smocks.

Another one you must check out is 'MBI' Master Beauty Instruments.

Mature skin

It loses elasticity and its ability to retain moisture. Signs of aging (fine lines, wrinkles, and sagging).

Cleanser:
- Antioxidant
- Preserve moisture

Toner:
- Oxygenating toner
- Import minerals/nutrients to stimulate tired skin
- Enriches & nourishes
- Removes all surface impurities

Scrub:
- Almond & mineral
- Stimulates & oxygenates with paprika
- Ground ivy tones and tightens pores.

Masque:
- Firmness
- Battles free radicals
- Stimulate & cleanse to rejuvenate and refine
- Increase collagen production
- Skin elasticity & texture
- Anti-wrinkle

Serum:
- Vit 'B & C' to strengthen & firm skin
- Boost moisture retention ability
- Resistance to environmental factors
- Tone and moisturize
- Lift facial contours & treat signs of aging due to menopause, breakouts, hormonal imbalances & collagen loss

- Plump up loss of skin tone

Moisturizer:

- Tone & firm skin
- Nourish & enrich, raising moisture levels to reduce signs of aging
- Moisturize
- Rejuvenate
- Minimize fine lines
- Antioxidant

***

Here is a fun mask to try... it is called the

**'Phyto 5 Element Mask,'
by Swiss Natural Energetic Skincare**

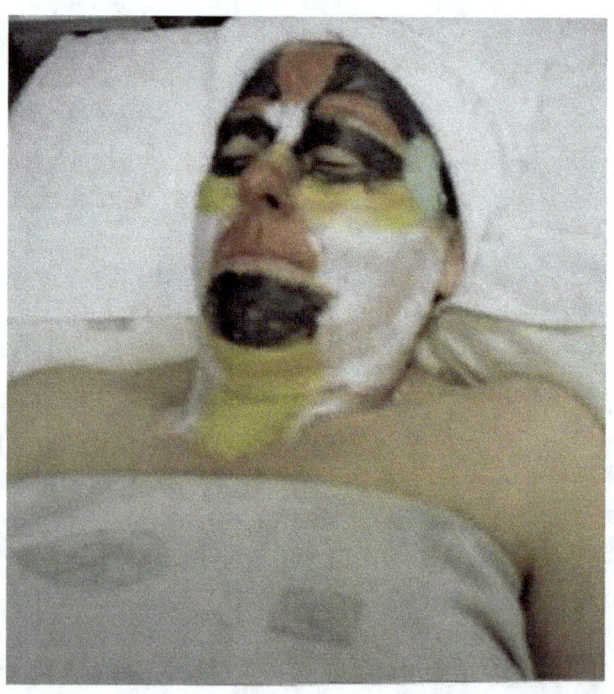

Dry Skin

    Cleanser:

- Hydrating
- Preserve moisture

    Toner:

- Import minerals/nutrients to stimulate
- Enriches & nourishes
- Removes all surface impurities

    Scrub:

- Almond & mineral
- Stimulates & oxygenates with paprika

    Masque:

- Stimulate & cleanse to rejuvenate and refine
- Increase collagen production
- Skin elasticity & texture
- Anti-wrinkle

    Serum:

- Vitamin 'B & C' to strengthen & firm skin
- Boost moisture retention ability
- Resistance to environmental factors
- Moisturize

    Moisturizer:

- Nourish & enrich, raising moisture levels
- Moisturize
- Rejuvenate

More fun Masks to try...

Casmara sells premium grade peel-off masks, *(make sure the client's hair is tucked in and wipe the product off as it dries - it runs a bit by the ears)*. Put a throw away the cloth under their head and shoulders. Soooo, cool when you pull it off.

New Directions Aromatics sells wonderful powder masks that you can mix with hydrosol water and apply with a brush.

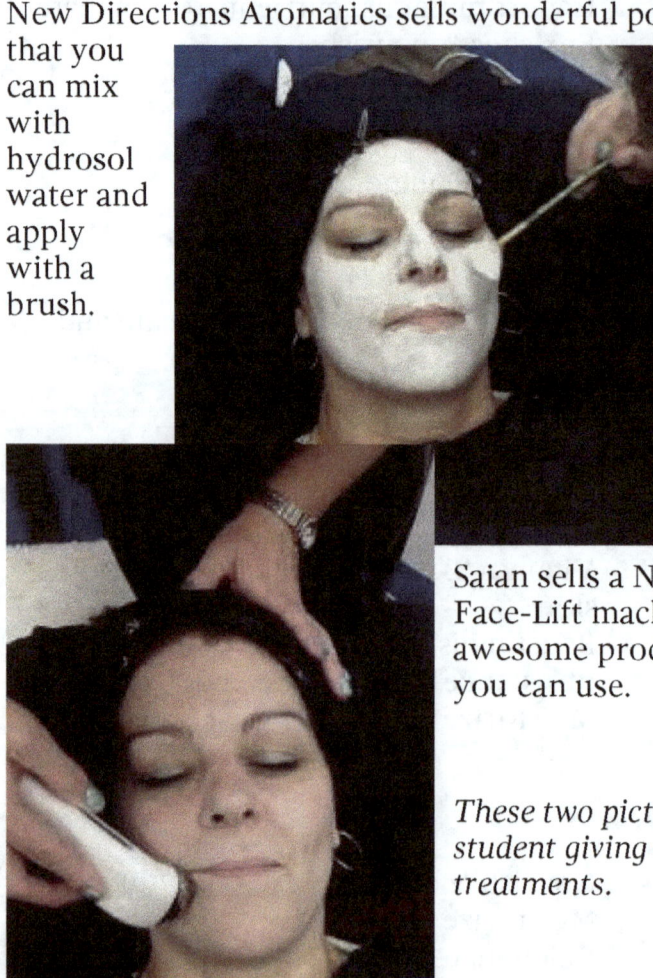

Saian sells a Non-Surgical Face-Lift machine and awesome products that you can use.

These two pictures are of a student giving me treatments.

COMMON SKIN DISORDERS

Acne

An inflammatory disease of the oil glands. Most prevalent in teenagers but common in adults as well.

Combination Skin

A combination of the symptoms of both dry and oily skin; most commonly consists of an oily

T-Zone area (around nose and forehead) and dry cheeks.

Comedo

A "blackhead". A "plug" of oil filling the pilosebaceous orifice, capped with blackened debris caused by oxidation.

Dehydrated Skin

A lack of moisture, which is often mistaken for dry skin yet can be present in all skin types; characterized by flakiness and fine lines.

Dermatitis

A general term for inflammation of the skin. A common form of this condition is Contact Dermatitis, which is the skin's reaction to an encounter with a specific allergen, i.e. Jewelry, make-up, fabrics, etc.

Dry Skin

> An under-functioning of the sebaceous glands, characterized by fine lines, coarse texture, and a dull appearance.

Eczema

> A generic term for acute or chronic inflammatory conditions which often include dryness and scaly skin, frequently accompanied by sensations of itching and or burning.

Milium

> A "whitehead" is a small deposit of keratin, covered by a thin layer of epidermal cells.

Oily Skin

> An over functioning of the sebaceous glands, distinguished by comedones, milia, and a shiny appearance.

Putstule

> Is a blemish containing pus.

Papule

> Is a solid blemish without the presence of pus.

Sensitive Skin

> Skin that readily reacts to a variety of factors such as specific chemicals, airborne debris, or certain skincare ingredients; symptoms include blotchiness, breakouts, or excessive dryness.

Set up for a Facial:

Depending on your place of employment and what products are carried in the spa, you will choose your product for your client first, then you will make the bed and lay out towels for her wrap and her face. If you use the crockpot method, you will fill it with water and turn it on high with your towels wet and rolled up.

You may burn some essential oil a diffuser or incense depending on the preference...you also will get your props ready.

As every establishment is different, this gives you a good guideline when you are lost or confused.

1. Cover a table with a clean towel or cloth to set your products on.
2. Choose your products depending on the client's skin type (if this is a new client, wait and do your consultation and look at their skin before choosing product). If you are only using the product for one skin type, make sure it is for sensitive skin. You can put enough products into individual containers or leave them in the original packaging. Make sure you always clean the bottles after each use.
3. Have two stainless silver or glass bowls; one small (to mix the mask in) and one large (to wring the hot towels in).
4. One facial fan brush to apply the mask
5. Cosmetic pads
6. Eye make-up removal

7. Little glass dish or pump bottle with massage oil in it.
8. One towel to wrap the head (if they have long hair use two; one you wrap around their head and the other you lay lengthwise covering the remainder of hair).
9. Bobby pin or hair clip (used to fasten the ends of the towel on their forehead)
10. Make the massage table up with a single sheet set; if it is cold, put a blanket on top. Fold back part of the sheet so the client can easily tell the bottom sheet.
11. Have a pillow for the head and ask if they need one for their knees.
12. In the crockpot, place six rolled up hand towels. Cover with water and heat (make sure when you use them to wring out all the water). You can use a kettle of hot water and a bowl to wet the towels. Have a container of cold water nearby in case you need to cool down the towels. The temperature of the towels should not ever burn them. If you cannot touch the towels, it is too hot for their face.
13. Have a robe or warp waiting in the room as well just in case they must go to the washroom.

Facial Procedure

1. Prepare room
2. Greet the client; Do the client consultation — check if any allergies and check skin type.
3. <u>Tell</u> the client what she or he needs to do to get ready for the facial:
   a. Remove any make-up, eye make-up, and jewelry.
   b. To get undresses when you leave the room, she needs to remove her shirt a bra at least (or drop the straps down her arms).
   c. To get under the covers on the massage table facing up.
   d. That you will knock on the door before coming back in.
4. Take off <u>your</u> jewelry and sanitize your hands (make sure your nails are not too long).
5. Wait at least three to four minutes and then knock on the door before you re-enter the room. You can turn down the lights and turn on some music. *I usually tell them what I am doing, so I do not surprise them.*
6. Towel the client's hair. They should have no hair showing around the face.
   a. Twist stared

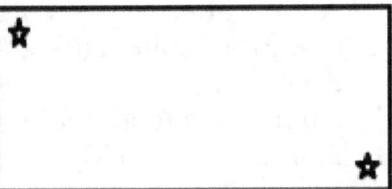

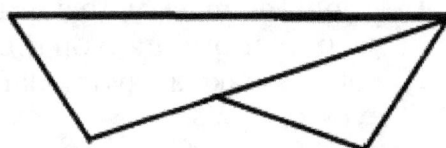

end to become the triangle parts.
   b. Lay the client's head on the straight end, just at the base of the hairline.
   c. Bring straight end together and hold in place with a hair clip.
   d. Tuck loose ends into the towel.
   e. If needed, use a second towel to cover long hair flowing out.
   f. Check the client's face, and then choose your products (if need be, go and get what you need – sometimes you will know ahead of time and get ready just as the client comes into the spa).

7. Product Procedure:
   a. Apply **cleanser** to both sides of your fingers and then begin by placing the back of your hand on client's forehead (this just warns them that you are starting), then work your way from the décolletage (shoulder/neck) up. (See the page following of the face pictures); do each of the steps on the picture three times (you do have a choice to do each three times or do the sequence three times).
   b. **Remove** cleanser with a hot towel.
   c. Apply **toner** to two cotton pads (one for face, one for décolletage); apply, starting at the décolletage.
   d. Apply the **facial peel or scrub** and work (page 2 of face pictures).
   e. **Remove** peel/scrub with hot towels
   f. Apply **toner**
   g. Apply the **mask** with a brush (you can place cucumber or potato on their eyes if you like). Potatoes take away the darkness under the eyes.
      h. Set timer for the required amount of time 10-20 minutes. (20 min. for mud)

      i. Do an arm and hand massage while the mask is drying.
      j. **Remove** the mask using hot towels.
      k. Prepare facial oil/cream for **massage** as if your client wants to be stimulated or relaxed. Then add essential oils.
      l. Undo the towel on the client's head and do a **scalp/hair massage**.
      m. End with a sweep of their hair, starting at their forehead and ending at the end of their hair.
8. If the client is asleep, touch their shoulder lightly, tell them quietly that the session is over, and once they are dressed to open the door so you know they are finished or to meet you in the lobby/front etc.
9. Offer them a drink of water when they come out.
10. Payment options: you might walk them to the till to pay and say goodbye you have office staff that handles that. Or some clients would rather pay beforehand so they can leave and enjoy the bliss of being pampered.
11. Clean up the room and prepare for the next client. The health board requires that everything you touch to be cleaned or wiped with antibacterial cleanser (after washing, spray all tools, bowels etc. with a mixture of equal parts water and rubbing alcohol).
12. <u>Tips are not mandatory</u> for any client to leave. If they do leave you a tip, thank them. Sometimes the client leaves a tip in the room, so you will not know they have tipped you until after they have left.

The facial should take about one hour.

Tips and tricks of Massage Manipulations, and Techniques

Every facial session will combine one or more of these basic movements. Each manipulation is applied in a definite way for a particular purpose. It is used according to the clients' condition and the desired result. The result of a session will depend on the amount of pressure, the direction of the movement, and the duration of each type of manipulation.

The usual direction of facial manipulation is from the insertion of a muscle to its origin.

> The origin of a muscle is the fixed attachment of one end of that muscle to a bone or tissue.
>
> The insertion is the attachment of the opposite end of the muscle to another muscle, or to a movable bone or joint.

Caution:

> Massaging a muscle in the wrong direction (from its origin to insertion) could result in the loss of resiliency and the sagging of the skin and muscles.

Types of Movements

Effleurage (stroking movement)

Effleurage is a light and continuous movement applied with the fingers and palms in a slow and rhythmic gliding manner. No pressure is used. The palms are used over large surfaces, while the cushions of the fingertips are used over the small surfaces (around the eyes).

Effleurage is frequently applied to the forehead, face, scalp, back, shoulders, neck, chest, arms, and hands for a soothing and relaxing effect.

Position of the fingers for stroking:

Curve the fingers slightly, with just the cushions of the fingertips touching the skin. Do not use the end of' the fingertips (nails) for massage movements. Fingertips cannot control the amount of pressure. In addition, free edges of the fingernails are likely to scratch the skin.

Positions of palms for stroking:

> Hold the whole hand loosely, keep the wrist and fingers flexible, and curve the fingers slightly to conform to the shape of the area being massaged.

Petrissage (Kneading movement)

Petrissage:

Grasp the skin and flesh between the fingers and palm of the hand. As the skin is lifted from the face, squeeze, roll, or pinch with a light, firm pressure. This movement invigorates the part being treated and is usually limited to back, shoulder, and arms.

Kneading:

The pressure should be light but firm. When grasping and releasing the fleshy parts, the movements must be in rhythm, never jerky. Kneading movements give deeper stimulation to the muscles, nerves, and skin glands, and improve circulation. Limited to the back, shoulder, and arms

Digital Kneading:

The cheeks can be massaged using a light pinching movement.

Fulling:

A form of petrissage is used when massaging the arms. With the fingers of both hands grasping the arm, a kneading movement is applied over the flesh. The kneading movement must be used with light pressure on the underside of the client's forearm, and between the shoulder and elbow.

Friction (Deep rubbing movement)

Friction:

This movement requires pressure on the skin while it's being moved over the underlying structures. Use your fingers or palms. Friction has a marked influence on the circulation and glandular activity of the skin. Hands move in opposite directions.

Circular friction movements:

Are usually used on the scalp, arms, and hands. Light circular movements are usually used on the face and neck.

Chucking, rolling, and wringing:

Are variations of friction and are used principally to massage the arms and both legs.

The rolling movement

Requires that the tissues be compressed firmly against the bone and twisted around the arm or leg both hands of the practitioner are active as the flesh is twisted down the arm in the same direction.

DETAILED FACIAL MASSAGE PROCEDURE

DECOLOTTE

1. Across the décolleté 6x. *Effleurage*
2. Around the shoulders to the pressure point in the shoulder joint. *Effleurage*
3. Down the back and up the neck vertebrae. *Effleurage*
4. Up the neck 3x. *Effleurage*
5. Slide up to the forehead (Splitting into 3 effleurage using an overlapping circle formation). *Effleurage*
6. Top forehead to the pressure point 3x.
7. Middle forehead to the pressure point 3x.
8. Bottom forehead to pressure point 3x.

EYES

9. Using your ring finger circle around the eyes 3x. *Effleurage*

CHEEKS

10. Circles on the zygomatic (cheekbone) up to the temple 3x. *Friction*
11. Circles on the middle cheek to the hollow pressure point then circle up to the middle ear pressure point 3x. *Friction*
12. Circles on the lower cheek to the bottom ear pressure point. 3x *Friction*

LIPS

13. Removing your left hand, circle around the lips using your ring finger. *Friction*

NECK

14. Circle down the platysma (neck) pulling up firmly on the sternocleidomastoid (either side of the throat). 3x. *Friction*

CHEST & BACK

15. First place your right hand under the back and then the left,
16. Circle across and out to the shoulder 3x. *Friction*
17. Down the back up to the neck vertebrae 3x. *Effleurage*

FACE

18. Slide up to the forehead.
19. With the ring and middle finger feather at the center of the forehead moving down to the right temple. *Friction*
20. Feather over towards the left temple. (Vibrate for a few seconds). *Vibration*
21. Now feather back towards the center, 3x. *Friction*
22. Using your ring finger firmly slide over the eyebrow and lightly under the eye walking on the nerve points at the bridge of the nose. *Friction*
23. Move around the eyes with small circles, down the cheekbone and walk up the nose to the pressure point. 3x. *Friction*
24. Using your ring finger slide to figure 8. (Between the thumb and middle finger) 6x. *Friction*
25. Feather the forehead again. 3x. *Friction*
26. Open palm strokes. 5x (Do not touch the nose). *Effleurage*

27. Starting with the right hand, then the left, grip the chin and pull towards the ears. *Petrissage (kneading)*
28. Middle finger around the lips. *Friction*
29. Lip pull with thumb and index fingers. 3x (Both hands). *Friction*
30. Chin pulls. 3x *Friction*
31. Circle down the platysma and up the sternocleidomastoid. 3x. *Friction*
32. Feathering from the chin to the shoulders. 3x (Each Shoulder). *Friction*

BACK
33. Down the arms. 3x   Effleurage
34. Back. 3x   Effleurage

FACE
35. Up the neck 3x, sliding the pinkie fingers to the base of the jaw on the last one *Friction*
36. Transfer your thumbs to the eyebrows
37. Slide across the brow stopping at the temple, with the thumb slide up between the eyes 3x *Friction*
38. Chin slaps – left side up to the lip – then right up to the lip – 3x. *Tapotement*
39. Feather upward on the left cheek then right cheek (Palm stroke over hand 2.5x). *Friction*
40. V's on forehead stopping at the temple (soft down hard up) 3x. *Friction*
41. V's on the cheek (Top to bottom) stopping at the pressure points 3x *Friction*
42. V's on the lower masseter region 3x *Friction*

CONCLUSION OF THE MASSAGE

43. Slide hands to décolletage, gentle strokes with flat hands across chest 6x. *Effleurage*
44. Back.
45. Neck 3x
46. Slide all fingers up to the forehead. *Effleurage*
47. Head press slide back towards you and slide to pressure points.
48. (Keep your pinkies on the client's face while sliding back)
49. Cup over eyes – hold
50. Slowly lightly feather off. *Friction*
51. Gently massage the head, slowly release the hair

Cleanser Application & Technique (do movements 3x)

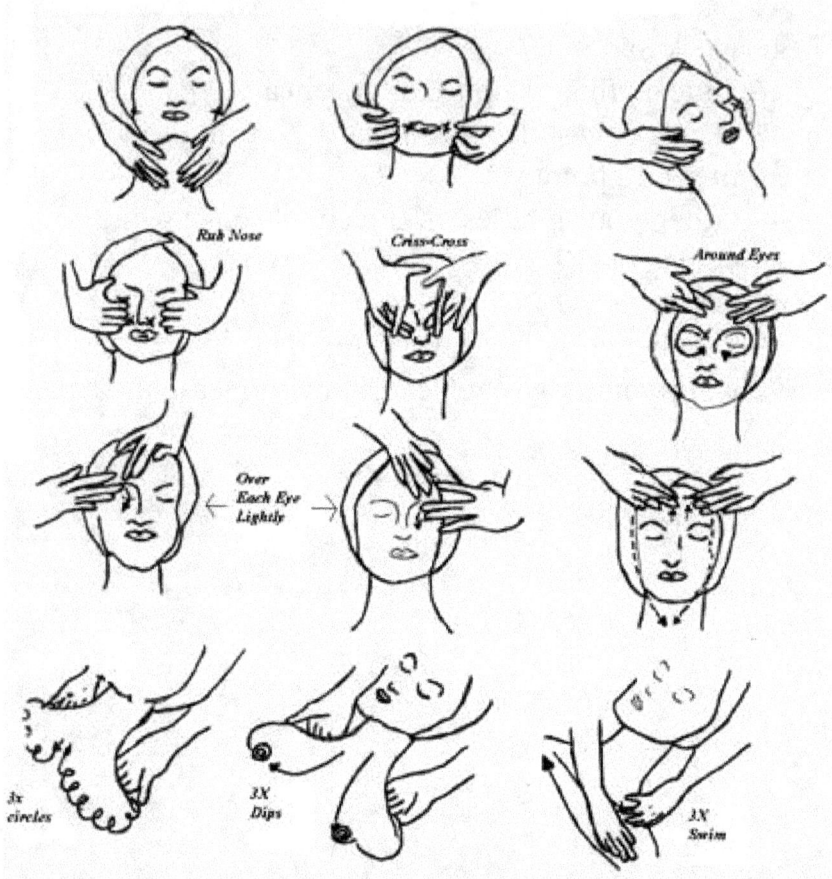

Toner Technique (do once after each procedure)

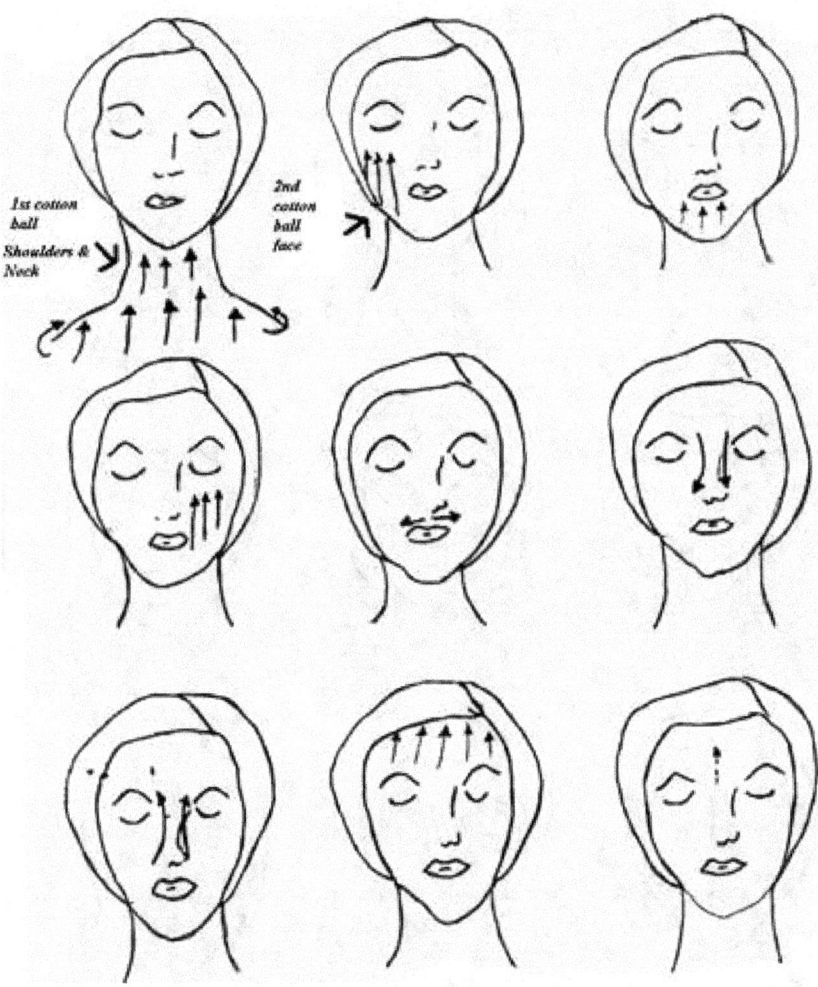

Scrub & Peel Technique (do 3x)

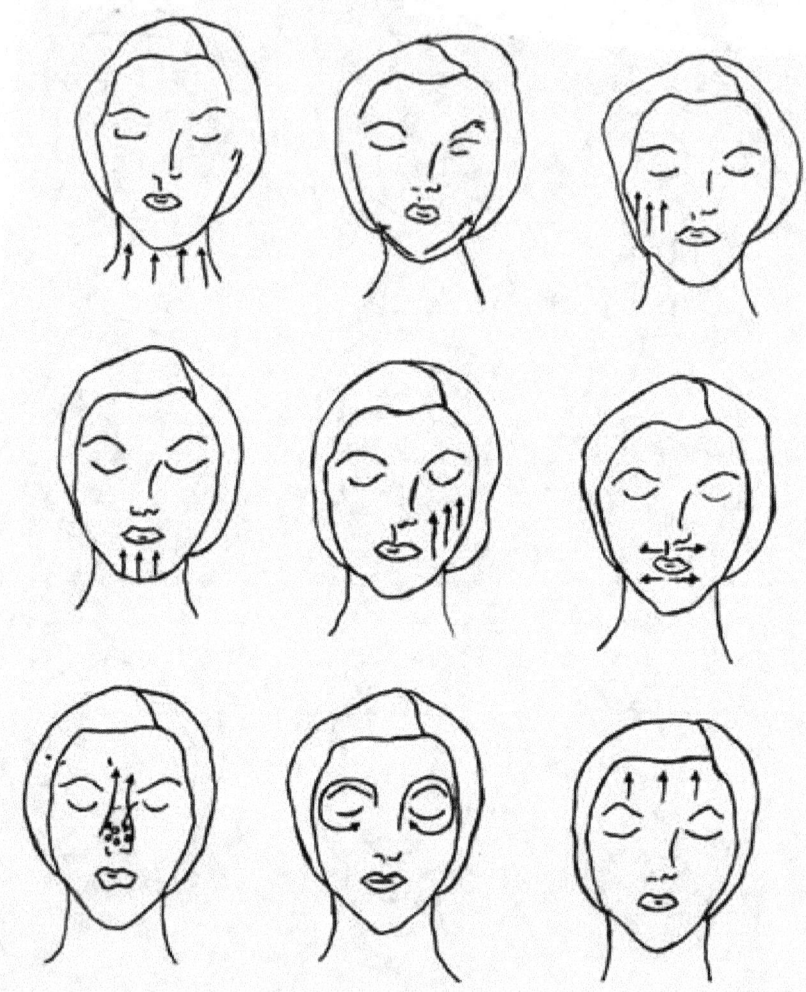

Remember to tone after you clean the product off!

Apply Mask Technique

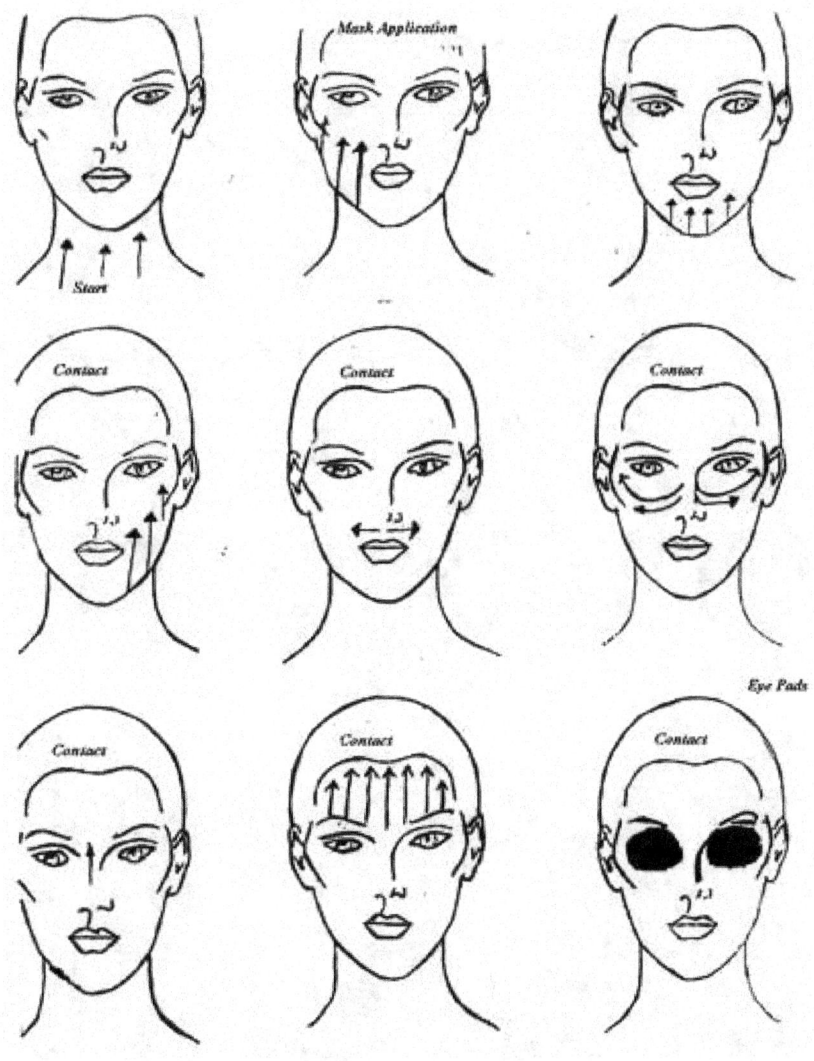

Remember to tone after you clean the product off!

Massage Technique (some estheticians do this before the mask procedure)

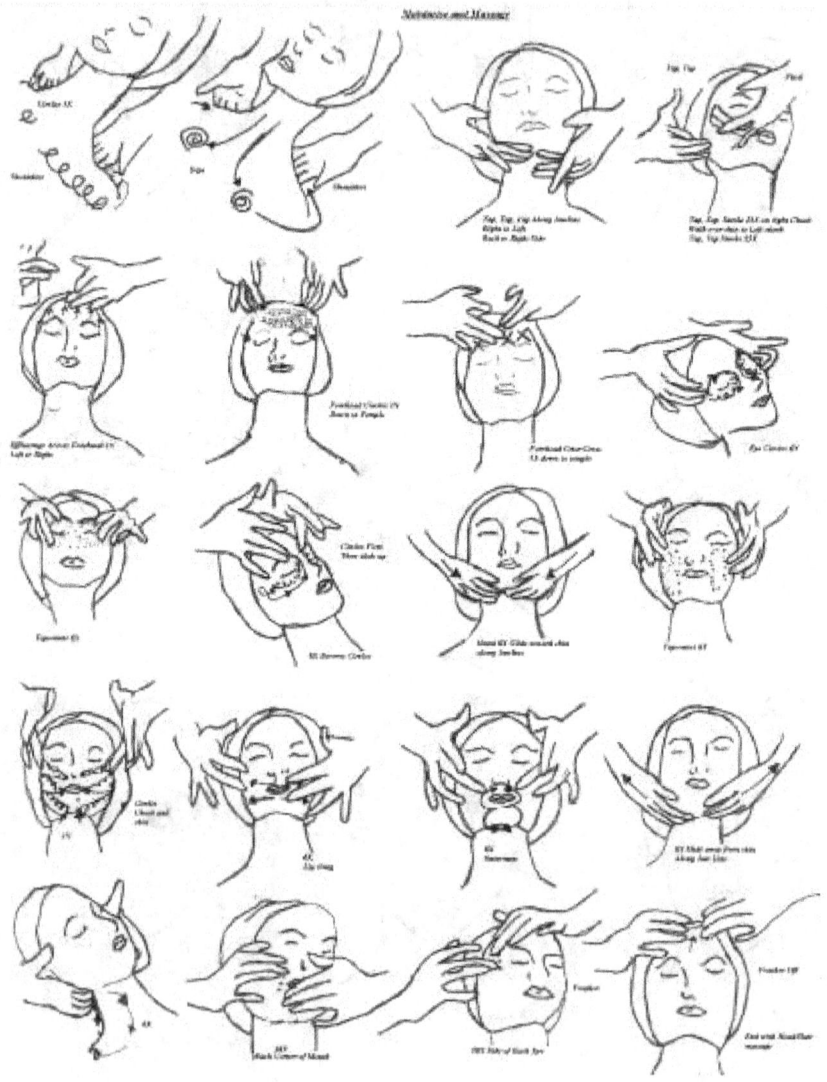

ADVANCED FACIAL PROCEDURE

1. (If using a Vapazone machine, turn it on until it starts to steam and then turn it off).
2. Cleanse
3. Remove and rinse with towel or sponge 3x (turn on steamer)
4. Tone
5. Gibson or Kleenex (Blot face)
6. Compress with towel 3x or Vapazone. (3-25 mm. Sensitive to Acneic)
7. (Gibson if needed)
8. Extractions.
    a. Begin with the nose, cheeks, chin, and forehead. (Move in a straight line, and then you will remove the sebum)
9. Tone (just the extracted areas)
10. Massage, use oil
11. (Rinse if needed, to remove excess oil)
12. Mask application using a brush (leave on for __?__ minutes) (crosswise)
13. Remove -apply hot compresses to loosen the mask and rinse with towel or sponge 3x
14. Gibson if needed
15. Tone
16. Moisturize the face and neck (tap to encourage absorption)
17. Eye serum if needed, lightly tap on under eye)
18. (If using a Hi-frequency machine, apply now).

Bonus Info for Facials

WOODS LAMP

Color	Issue
Bluish /white-	normal skin
White fluorescent- layer /aged	thick corneum
White Spots- cells (check if lint)	clump of dead
Purplish/blue violet- (usually nose)	dehydrated
Yellow/orange/pink-	oily skin (fat)
Shades of Purple/Gray/Brownish-	pigmentation
Reddish-	sensitive
Blue spots/shades of brown & white- texture)	mature (check

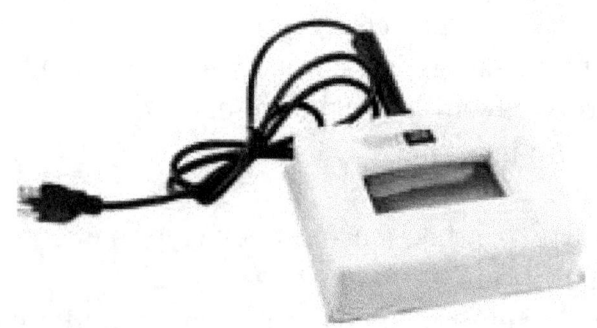

Excellent to use to see the true nature of the skin.

ACNE

Definitions:

Macule	< 1cm	flat (spot)
Patch	> 1cm	flat (spot)
Papule	< 1cm	elevated (like acne)
Plaque	> 1cm	extended solid
Nodule	> 1cm	Deeper solid
Vesicle (blister)	< 1cm	collection of free fluid
Bulla (blister)	> 1cm	collection of free fluid
Wheal		pus
Scale		epidermal thickening
Crust		dry serum
Fissure		crack or split
Erosion		loss of epidermis (scratch /no bleeding)
Ulcer		deeper loss of epidermis & dermis
Lichenification (mapping)		thickening of skin line
Scar		thickening of fibrous tissue
Atrophy		loss of substance (thinning)
Excoriation		linear erosion

Causes:

1) Juvenile   - Face

2) Digestive   - Forehead/upper back Treat liver

3) Hormonal   - Chin

Face cells change every 28 days

Grades of Acne:

<u>Grade 1</u>

- Open & closed comedones –blk heads & whiteheads

- No inflammatory lesions (leads to scars)

- Scarring unlikely

<u>Grade 2</u>

- Comedones

- Papules

- Few Pustules (lesions with yellowish pus cap appearance, blister)

<u>Grade 3</u>

- Comedones

- Papules

- Few Pustules

- Few nodules – small solid nodes (not visible touch only)

Grade 4 Refer to Dermatologist!

- Few comedones
- Some Papules
- Many Pustules
- Nodules
- Cysts

Metal Tools

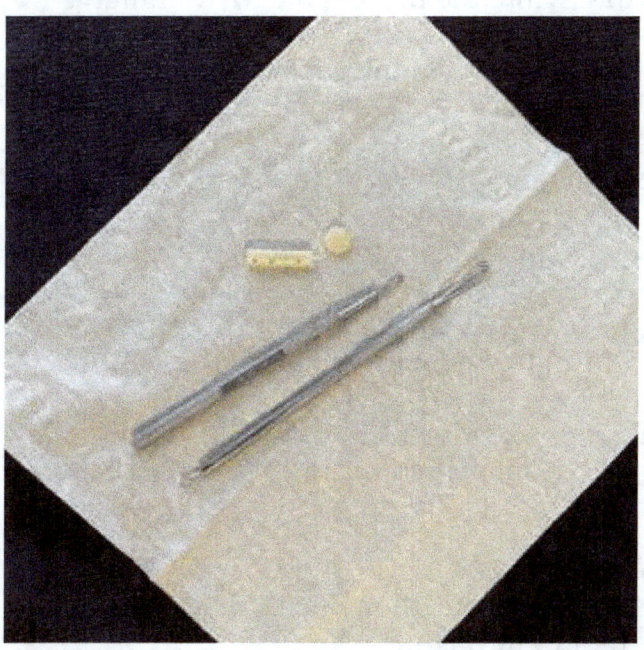

Sterile Lancet (pin on the end)
Ultra Comedo Extractors - Stainless Steel

If Using Hormeta Products

Change pillowcases daily

Clean phone, helmet, chairs etc. daily and No hair products

Procedure:

1. Cleanse (twice if wearing make-up)
2. Tone (anti-bacterial and PH
3. Discrustate –need to liquefy the skin, can use a mask (wheat/ bran enzyme or papaya), (can use a galvanic machine)
4. Steam – while the mask is on 10-15 minutes (not if using skin or oral products)
5. Remove with warm towels (not hot)
6. Let the skin rest for 1-2 minutes
7. Extraction (10 minutes max) (comedones and select pustules only)
    a. Acne lesions- (5x magnifying lens) press in and lift out in the direction of the hair growth. Do not squeeze!
8. High-Frequency machine (kills bacteria) (contra-indicated with metal or pregnancy)
9. Tone
10. Ampoules – optional
11. Mask – 10-minute sulfur mask
12. Hydrate

Do 1x/2x week for 6 weeks, then once every 3 weeks, then once per month until gone.

Home care:

Cleans 2x/day

Tone

Hydrate at night

-Do not exfoliate grade 3 acne skin!!

-The skin may still be purging even after 24 hours.

-Chronic skin issues cannot be fixed in ten minutes of exfoliation.

-Pore size (Cells) can shrink

If Using Moor Mud Treatment

-Apply the mask (can be done on the back also) (men two minutes only)

-Steam

-Remove

-Extractions

ELECTROTHERAPY

Microcurrent -

Amp –	unit of strength
Milliamperes-	1/1000th of an amp
Milliamperemeter-	is the instrument used to measure the electrical current
Volt-	unit of pressure (110 or 220)
Ohm-	unit of resistance
Watt-	measure of electricity used per second (40, 60, 100–eg. light bulbs)
Hertz (Hz)-	frequency

Electrotherapy uses special currents to create certain effects on the skin.

1. Galvanic-
    - Also known as ionization. Direct current of low volt and high amp.
    - Used to force water-soluble skincare products into the skin.
    - **Phoresis** -Galvanic current occurs when the current passes through particular **acid** (positively charged/ anode: P or + or red) or **alkaline** (negatively charged / cathode: N or – or black) solutions and/or by passing the current through the body tissues and fluids.
        - **Anaphorisis**-allows alkaline solution to enter the skin (negative pole of an electrode). Used with desincrustation- clogged pores or blackheads.
            - In desincrustation, an alkaline (**negative** charged) solution is applied to the skin. Electrode held

by practitioner is **negative**. These repel each other and force **alkaline** product **into the skin**
- In iontophoresis, an acid (**positive** charged) solution is applied to the skin. Electrode held by practitioner is **positive**. These repel each other and force **acid** product **into the skin**
- Always finish with the positive polarity.
  - Cataphoresis- allows an acid solution to enter the skin (positive pole of an electrode). Used in iontophoresis – deeper layers of the epidermis are built up or nourished.

-When the electrode held by the Esthetician is in the positive mode, the reaction on the skin is acidic.

- When the electrode held by the Esthetician is in the negative mode, the reaction on the skin is alkaline.

	Alkaline	Acid
Product	negative	positive
Practitioner	negative charged electrode	positive charged electrode
Client	positive charged electrode	negative charged electrode

2. High Frequency

- Oily skin with overall congestion. Formation of Ozone to produce germicidal effect

3. Faradic

- Produces a mechanical, non-chemical reaction; stimulates nerve and muscle tissue with current traveling through motor nerves between two positioned electrodes.

4. Sinusoidal

- Deeper then faradic

SILHOUET TONE -QUINTET FACIAL MACHINE

High Frequency: germicidal, stimulating, and soothing
Gently rotate the glass back and forth to insert into the machine

*Touch the glass and then the client

Large Mushroom Electrode: recommended for normal, oily & acne skin

Small Mushroom Electrode: recommended for normal, dry & sensitive skin

Cylindrical Electrode: recommended for all skin types (indirect massage or saturation)

Clean with Steraldex machine (UV)

- used for sterilizing equipment after wiping off with a soft tissue.

DO NOT USE ALCOHOL ON ELECTRODES
"as it will damage them!

Techniques:

Direct Contact:

>Use: Large glass mushroom   Intensity: 3-4

>Time: 4 minutes (Purchase egg timer)

>Make sure you touch & hold glass before touching client, once on then let go

>Gently glide it on the skin of the face

>Performed after extractions <u>or</u> after protection cream application to enhance cream's penetration.

Sparking:

>Use: Small glass mushroom   Intensity: 4-5
>   Time: 4 minutes

>Make sure you touch & hold glass before touching client, once on then let go

>Gentle "tapping" procedure with glass mushroom

>>Disinfects and stimulates the skin with direct contact on blemishes helping to destroy bacteria and promote healing. Use dry sterile gauze squares between acneic skin and electrode, thus producing ozone to help dry pustular infections, destroying germs and bacteria, thus promoting healing.

Indirect Massage:

>Use: Cylindrical Electrode Intensity: 0 to 1-2
>   Time: 4 minutes

>Removed ALL JEWELRY

The client holds Cylindrical Electrode with one hand

The practitioner uses a light tapping technique with fingers over wrinkles and face

> High frequency to increase cellular metabolism in very precise areas and increasing blood circulation.

Energizing Treatment:

Use: Cylindrical Electrode

Intensity: 0 to 1-2   Time: 5 minutes

Apply mask

The client holds the Cylindrical Electrode with one hand

Practitioner DO NOT TOUCH CLIENT

> Good for overworked, stressed, lack of energy, and induced alternating polarity current, which energizes the whole body resulting in an overall feeling of wellbeing.

Rotary Brushes:

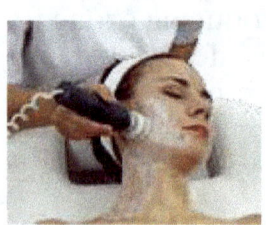

Use: Rotary Brushes Intensity: 6-7 Time: All face 3x

Use after make-up removal.

Soft bristle brushes are for the face

The firm brush is for the back and feet

Technique:

1. Apply foaming cleanser
2. Dampen brush and use light pressure with back and forth movement

Facilitates extractions and permits better absorption of active ingredients used

Spray Machine:

Use: Spray Machine   Intensity: 9   Time: All face

Cover client's shoulders and the area around the neck with towels

Can be used for:

- Treatment to remove cleanser, mask, and residue
- Occasionally use <u>during</u> mask process to dampen mask.
- Low intensity to soothe and tonify after mask removal

Vacuum Machines: Apply finger on suction on- finger off, suction off.

Comedone Suction Cup: (small opening -pencil lead size)

Use: Comedone Suction Cup   Intensity: 9
          Time: Acne

Prior to manual extraction

Use on blackhead comedones in the areas around the nose, chin, etc.

Anti-Wrinkle: -rectangular opening

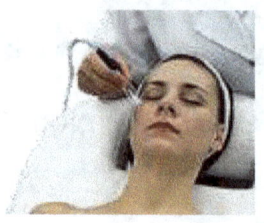

Use: Anti-Wrinkle

Intensity: 9	Time: Wrinkles

One hand holds the skin taut while other hand guide anti-wrinkle vacuum across individual wrinkles and lines

"X" pattern around eyes and mouth

Increases circulation, oxygenates skin & provides proper nutrition to the skin

Facial Massage Suction Cup: - bowl-shaped

Use: Facial Massage Suction Cup

Intensity: 3	Time: All face

Use before manual massage

Apply small amount lotion for a gliding effect

Increases circulation and provides better absorption of active ingredients

Galvanic Machine

Disincrustation: Liquefies grease and sebum (oily or t-zone areas only)

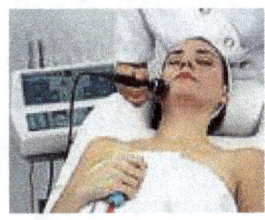

Use: Disincrustation

Intensity: .6 to 1.5 max (prickle feeling)   Time: 5 min

Solution: Water and 1% sodium bicarbonate

Use after make-up removal and before steaming face

Practitioner: using **BLACK WIRE** attachment machine Polarity is **negative**

- Blue sponge, fit into the black ring
- Wet blue sponge by dipping into a solution

Client: holding **RED WIRE** - is hand electrode client holds during the process

- Cover with wet blue pouch and cover with tissue for the client.

*Reverse polarity 1 min to balance PH

Iontophoresis Roller: - puts the product into the skin

Use: Iontophoresis roller

Intensity: 3   Time: 10 min

The metallic roller **must** be of the same polarity as the product being used.

Gauze is soaked with product and wrapped around the roller.

Glide lightly over skin, concentrating on fine lines and wrinkles.

Iontophoresis Pen: Wrinkles

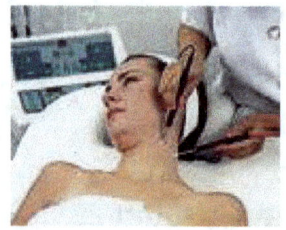

Use: Iontophoresis pen

Intensity: 3   Time: 3min

- to be used after anti-wrinkle suction cup
- apply the anti-wrinkle gel to cleansed skin (product must be the same polarity as the pen electrode)
- glide pen along each wrinkle slowly 2 to 3 times
    - followed with manual massage and mask

* If you do not know product polarity, you can still gain penetration by selecting the negative polarity button for 3 minutes and then follow by the positive button for 3 minutes**

ONLY USE EXCELLENT PRODUCTS!!! FEED THE SKIN. Not all products are to be used with machines.

SECRET OF A HEALER – MAGIC OF ESTHETICS

Facial	Manual / by hand	Machine	Product	Time	Intensity	Normal	Dry	Oily	Combination	Acne/Problem	Sensitive	Mature
Cleanser Remove- Makeup												
		Soft Rotary Brush light pressure	Foamy cleanser	All face	6-7	*	*	*	*			*
	Or Clean by hand		?				*	*	*	*	*	*
Remove Product												
Dry by hand	Remove by towels	Spray / pads	water	All face	9	*	*	*	*	*	*	*
			Towel / Kleenex									
Wrinkles 2-3x on each wrinkle		Galvanic – Iontophoresis & hand held wet / Kleenex	? soap Same polarity as machine	10 min	0 to 10.3 max	*	*	*	*	*	*	*
		Roll										
		Galvanic – Pen & hand held wet / Kleenex	Gel	Polarity same 6 min 3 min + 3 min +	0 to 10.3 max	*	*	*	*	*	*	*
		Glide										
		HF-Cylindrical		All face Wrinkles	0 to 1-2	*	*	*	*	*	*	*
		Vacuum-Anti-wrinkle		Wrinkles	3x							
Extractions- Before												
		Vacuum – comedones		All acne	9	*	*	*	T-zone	*		
		Soft Rotary Brush (LP)	Peel cream	All face	6-7	*	*	*	*	*		*
High Frequency (HF) Lrg Mushroom		Direct Contact / glide		4 min	3-4	*		*	*	*		
HF Lrg Mushroom		Sparking / tapping Hold clean head with hand		4 min	4-5				gauze	*		
HF Sm Mushroom		Direct Contact / glide		4 min	3-4	*					*	

Facial	Manual / by hand	Machine	Product	Time	Intensity	Normal	Dry	Oily	Combination	Acne/Problem	Sensitive	Mature
	Exfoliate		Spa scrub	All face		*	*	*	*	Not level 3-4	*	*
		Galvanic – Disincrustation Neg-blk wire Pos-red wire glide	? or water & 1% sodium bicarbonate	5 min Reverse polarity 1 min PH	0.6 to 1.5			Oily	* Area only	*		
Steam	Towel or	Steamer	water	Before & during		?	*	?	*	*	?	?
	Extractions hand tool			All face				?	*	*	?	?
Remove Product	Remove by towels or	Spray /pads	water	All face	9	*	*	*	*	*	*	*
Massage	BY Hand		Cream	All face		*	*	*	*	*	*	*
	Follow with manual massage	1st Vacuum – suction cup	cream	5 min	3	*	*	*	*		*	*
	Remove by towels or	Spray /pads	water		9	*	*	*	*	*	*	*
Mask	By Hand		Mud or clay			*	*	*	*	*	*	*
	By hand or	HF – Cylindrical For product penetration DO NOT TOUCH CLIENT	Brush on ? (not mud or clay)	5 min	0 to 2-3	*	*	*	*	*	*	*
Remove Product	Remove by towels or	Spray /pads	water	All face	9	*	*	*	*	*	*	*
Tone	By hand	Spray	?	All face	?	*	*	*	*	*	*	*
Protector cream	By hand		Mild Aroma blend	All face		*	*	*	*	*	*	*
		HF by mushroom	?	All face	3-4	*	*	*	*	*	*	*
		HF – Cylindrical DO NOT TOUCH CLIENT	Protection cream	5 min	0 to 2-3	*	*	*	*	*	*	*

Make-Up

People have a favorite part of their face...

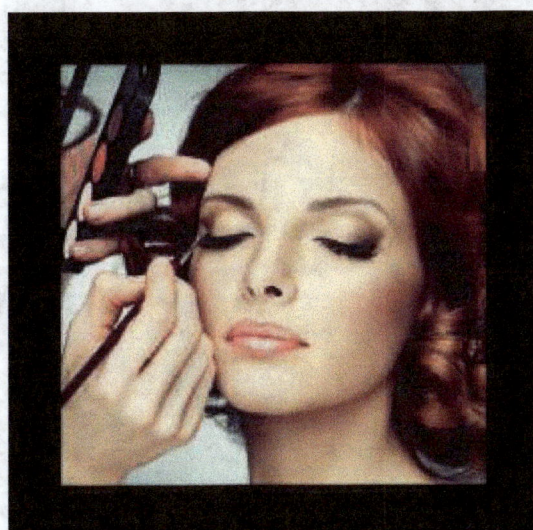

Usually, it is their eyes or lips, but it may be their brows or cheeks.

They also have something they do not like, their nose, mole, ears. It may even be their eyes or lips.

Find out what they like and don't like.

Questions to ask the client-

Are they...?

- When getting photos taken (lots of make up for good looking pictures)
    - Going out for a special occasion
    - Wedding
    - Grad
- First note client's style, they need to feel comfortable
    - light make-up
    - night make-up
    - Glitter and sparkle
    - Color of their liking.

Brushes

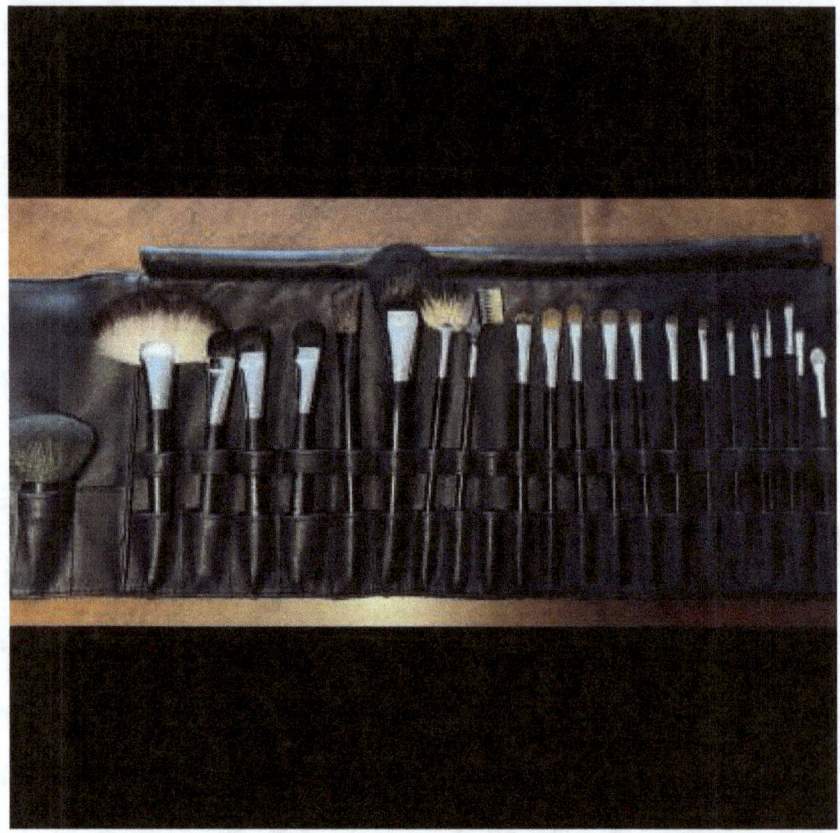

- Large Powder Brush – for applying loose, pressed, or bronzing powders, all over the face or where needed (from left – 1st and 2nd brush)
- Blusher Brush – next biggest brush, for applying blush to your cheeks (from left – 3rd–7th brushes – 6th is an angled blush brush)
- 3rd- 5th can be used as concealer brushes
- 8th is a fan brush – used for applying highlighter (I use it to apply face masks)

- 9th is a two-sided brow and comb brush, to shape your brows
- 10th is a small contour brush
- 11th-14th are straight, curved, and angled eye powder brushes
- 15th-18th are straight, curved, and angled eyeliner brushes
- 19th & 20th are lip liner brushes
- 21st is a shadow sponge brush

You can also purchase smudger brushes, they have a sponge at the tip and mascara wands.

The more hair on the brush, the more product it will hold.

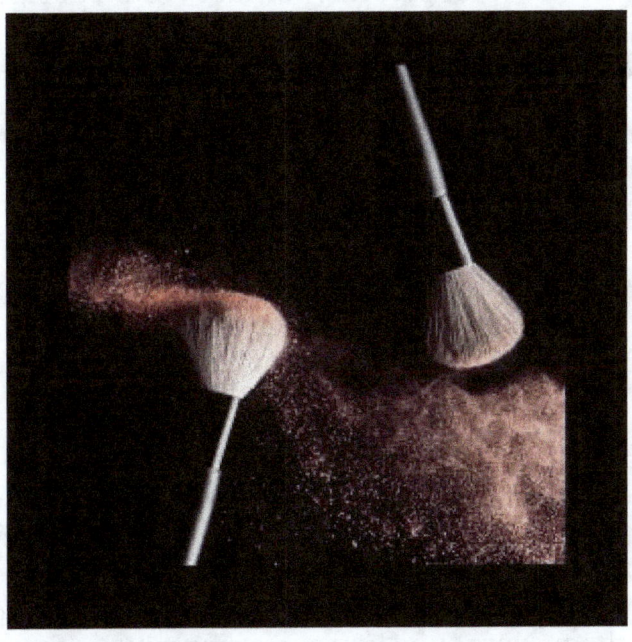

1st Step - what 'Shape' of face do they have?

1. Rectangle
2. Square
3. Triangle
4. Diamond
5. Inverted Triangle
6. Circle
7. Oval

The shape of face you are trying to achieve is oval.

To view your own face, look into a mirror and imagine there are dots in these locations...

- At the center of your forehead (at the hairline)
- Each side of your forehead (at the hairline)
- At the widest part of your face, your cheeks, and jaw
- And the center of your chin, and the lowest parts of your chin

What shape does the dots make?

Beautiful people have a synergistic flow to their faces.

For perfect synergy, an equal shape and size on both sides of the face and the distance between the top of the forehead to top of the eyebrows, top of the eyebrows to bottom of the nose, and bottom of the nose to the bottom of the chin are equally divided into three portions.

When you look at a person, your gaze should flow not get stuck at any one part. We star at people with synergy faces. Many actors and actresses have make-up artists creating the illusion of perfect synergy so that we love to look at them. Next time you see a magazine at the grocery store that shows before and after make-up of an actress, take a good look... there are some fantastic make-up artists out there!

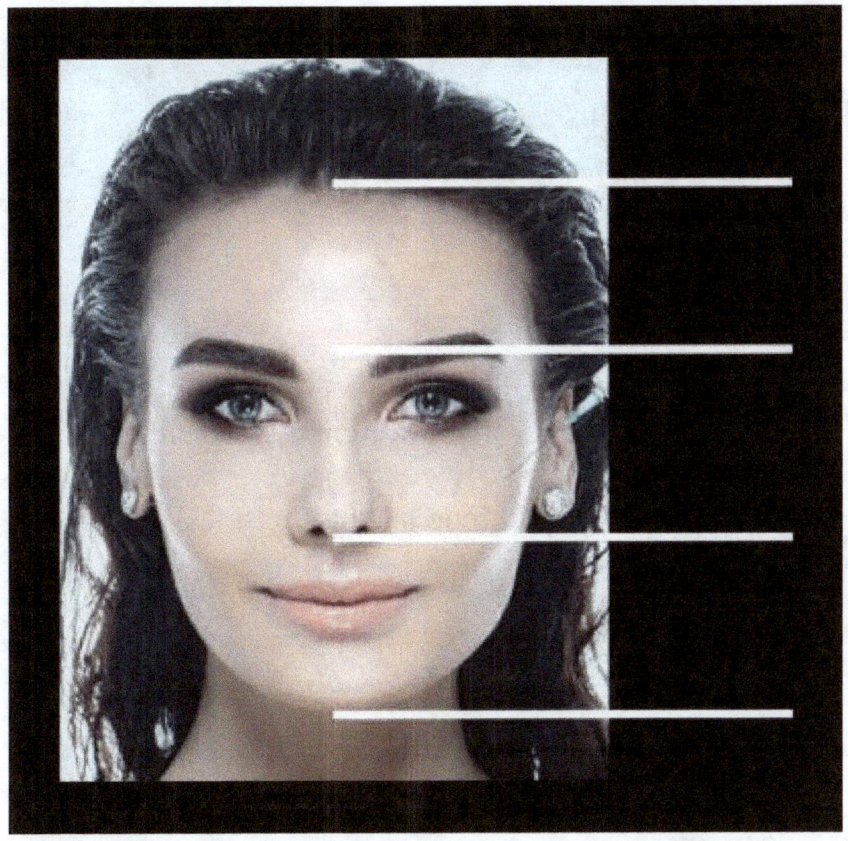

Here you can see that her brows are too high. She has a rectangle face but notice the make-up shading from the nose down, and by the eyes, it gives an oval illusion.

Most faces have a high side and low side of face; check both ears, brows, and corner of the mouth.

- Always do the make up to the high side.

2nd and 3rd Steps

Secrets to Concealer Colors

4 different ways to use light

    1. Reflecting

    2. Highlighting

    3. Fill in

    4. Counter shading

Color corrects in the same way as the need.

- For a pimple use a dot (a pimple is a dead cell and is grey/red)
- Any groove or indent is light/the sides are shadow
- Break the line
- Blend
- Correct spot
- If you want any area fuller – add color

Basic Color Chart

- ✓ Red - use green
- ✓ Orange- use turquoise (standing in a pool everyone looks good).
- ✓ Gold/yellow- use blue
- ✓ Yellow/green- use violet
- ✓ (Using complementary color will balance/neutralize it. Look at their wrist for their true color)
- ✓ You can blend colors to create the ideal color for their complexion.

*At the end of putting on the make-up check if you need to re-apply to any pimpled areas.

I had a student once who was a professional make-up artist, and she said that she has a palette of over thirty colors and shades for contour and concealer use.

Tips to remember:

- Red- tightens and empowers structure
- White- shows undertone color
- Volume = height, width & depth
- Menstruating changes the color of a person's skin.
- Oxidizes - deeper white
- The color needs to be applied in 3 places to look natural
- Concealer works for still photos, not for moving people in the film industry or real life.
- Movement- in the face, all muscles are attached at one end only.
- Did you know to remove yellow stains from a white cloth, instead of using bleach, use liquid blue product.

Did you know? Grocery stores use color to enhance a product. Meat is wrapped in colored plastic (blue, violet, or yellow) to make meat look redder.

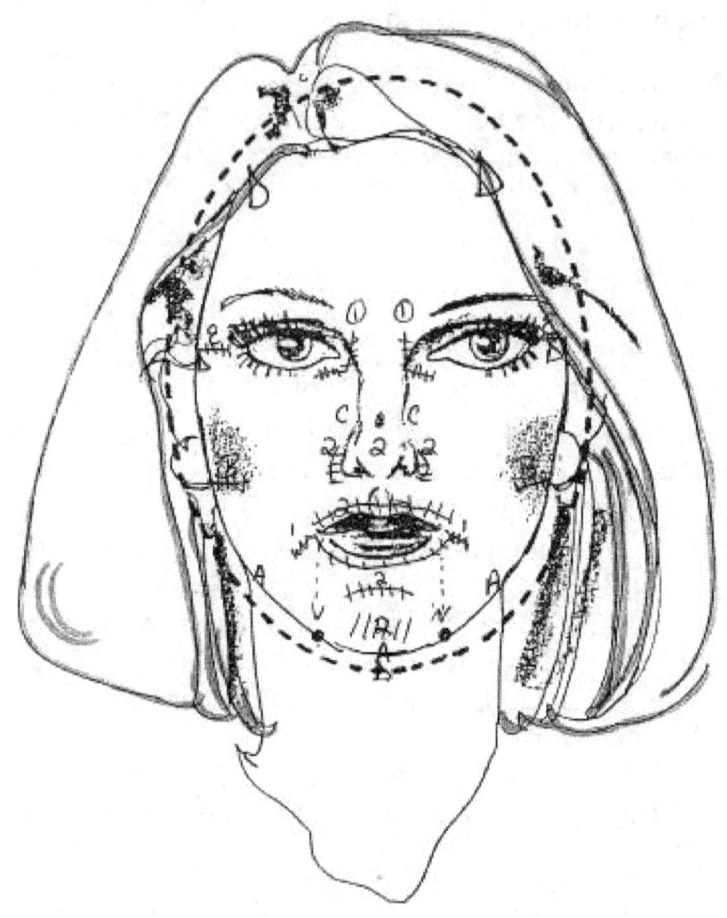

Follow this picture when applying concealer

(Loved what I originally learned through Keyano Aromatics!)

Secrets to Counter Shading Colors

This **IS NOT** the same as foundation, cover-up, or concealer!

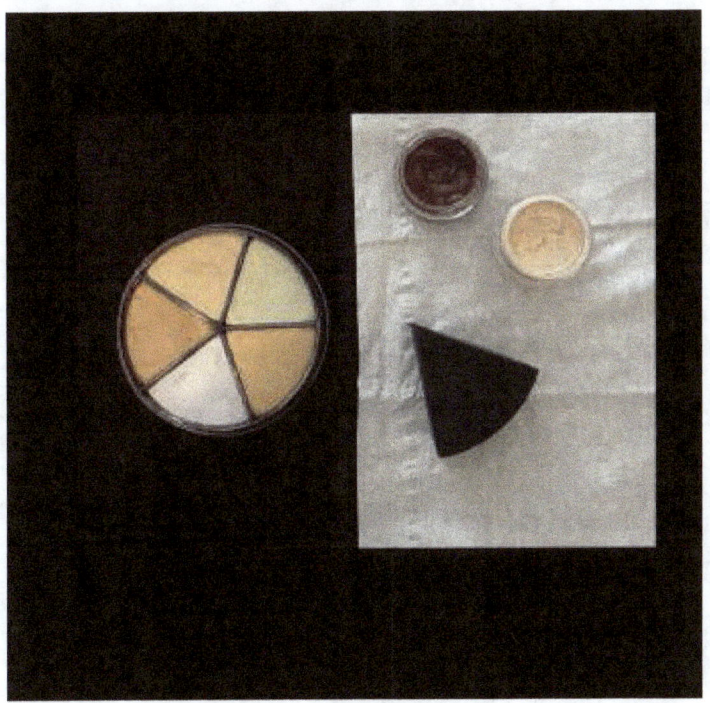

Product on the left is concealer, two on top are contour colors (and a triangle sponge for blending)

Counter Shading is different than concealer...

- Concealer – covers a blemish and creates an even color to the skin
- Counter shading uses the product on the shadow areas of the face
- Always counter shade on the area of the face that does not move.

1. Ivory or Light concealer - (brings things forward/closer) covers scars indents and dark circles. (can be used over dark or green)
2. Dark Beige or Dark contour – shape and define

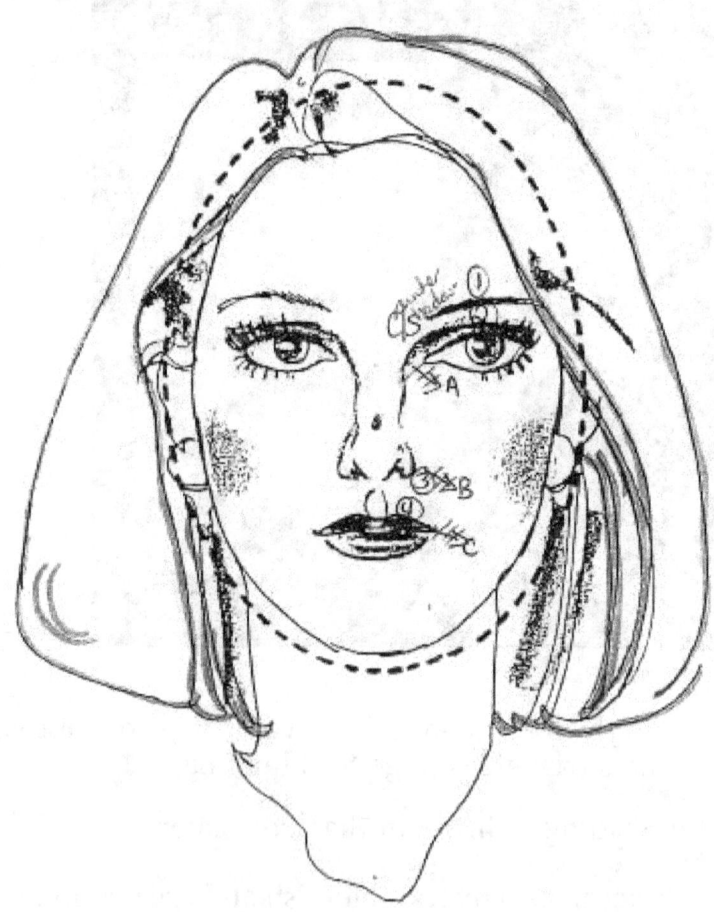

Follow this picture when counter shading

4th Step – Foundation

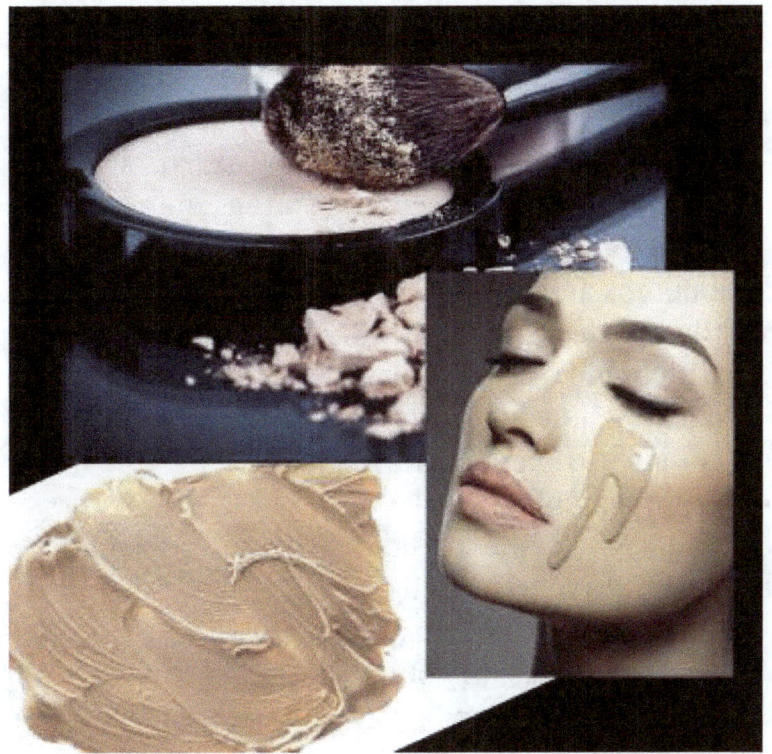

Some professionals do this step before the concealer.

Foundation Rules for a Beautiful Complexion:

- Start with a clean canvas, having a facial, or at least exfoliating every couple of weeks should do the trick.
- Hydrate your skin with moisturizer before applying make-up. Let it dry fully!

- Many professionals use a Primer, it is a preparatory product that is applied after your skincare to create an ideal canvas to hold onto whatever make-up comes afterward — like foundation, tinted moisturizer, or concealer. Your primer might come in the form of a hyaluronic acid-spiked facial serum that boosts hydration, a sunscreen that protects and softens the appearance of pores, or a traditional silicone-based primer that smooths and blurs.
- Choose the right formula. Drier skin works best with liquid or cream formulas, whereas combination and oily skins can handle stick, compact, or powder formulations.
- Color matching!!!
    - The color should match your skin color.
    - Not darker or lighter!!!
    - When choosing a shade, try three close matches on your jawline, and choose the one you can hardly see.
    - You may need more than one color as the seasons' change
- Blend, blend, and blend again. No edges of where the color starts of finishes should be visible
- Seal in the liquid foundation by using a no color powder over the top.
- Maintenance, a pressed powder is great for touch-ups when you start to look shiny (hot summer day will do that to a girl).
- Never EVER sleep ion your foundation, your skin needs to breathe!

Cheeks

You make me Blush... In the old days, they pinched their cheeks for color.

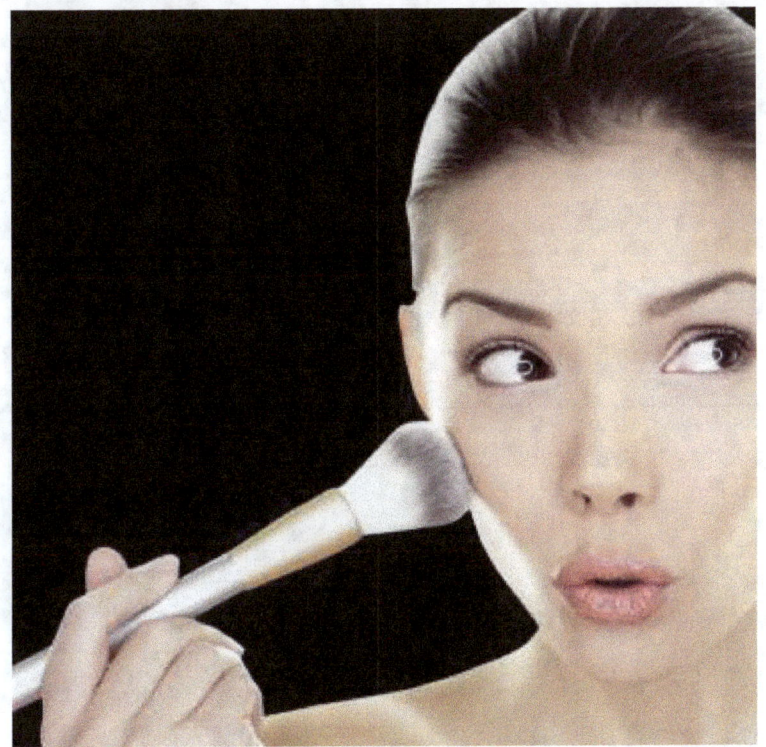

Pretty much, there are three choices:

1. Inside corner – from the hairline, angled to the corner of your lip and stopping at the inside of your pupil (closest to your nose)
2. Center Pupil - from hairline, angled to corner of your lip, and stopping at the center of your pupil
3. Outside corner - from the hairline, angled to the corner of your lip and stopping at the start of your pupil (closest to your ear)

Most professionals start at the hairline and brush towards the nose, but for more color, you can start the other way.

Lips

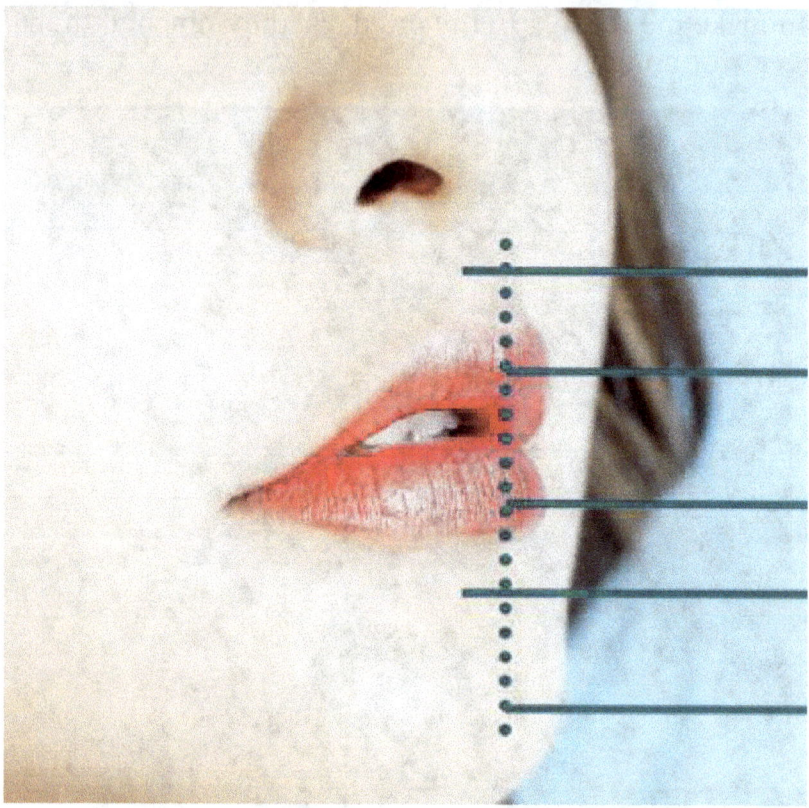

- The top lip, bottom lip, and chin should each extend equally.
- The areas above and below the lip should indent
- The bottom lip should be fuller than the top lip
- The outside corners of the mouth should turn slightly up, and end at the start the inside of each pupil
- The 'cupids bow' should be the highest point to the mouth

Tone & Blood

Lack of color is a lack of activity.
- Nutrition- how you like to eat.
- verbalization- how you express
- sexuality- red lips
- When you are excited physically, your lips will change color.
- Use peach lipstick on oily skin people to make red.

You can create the illusion of bigger or smaller lips by using a lip pencil.

- Draw a line above the natural lip line for a fuller look,
- or inside the natural lip line for a thinner look.
- Using a lip pencil helps the lipstick color from bleeding.

You can put concealer or foundation on your lips to change the shape and color.

Eyes

Perfect eyes are

- 2/3 from the bottom of the eyebrow to the crease above the eye
- 1/3 from the crease above the eye to the corner of the eye
- Eyes are spaced with the same size as the real eye (inside corner to the other inside corner – across the nose)

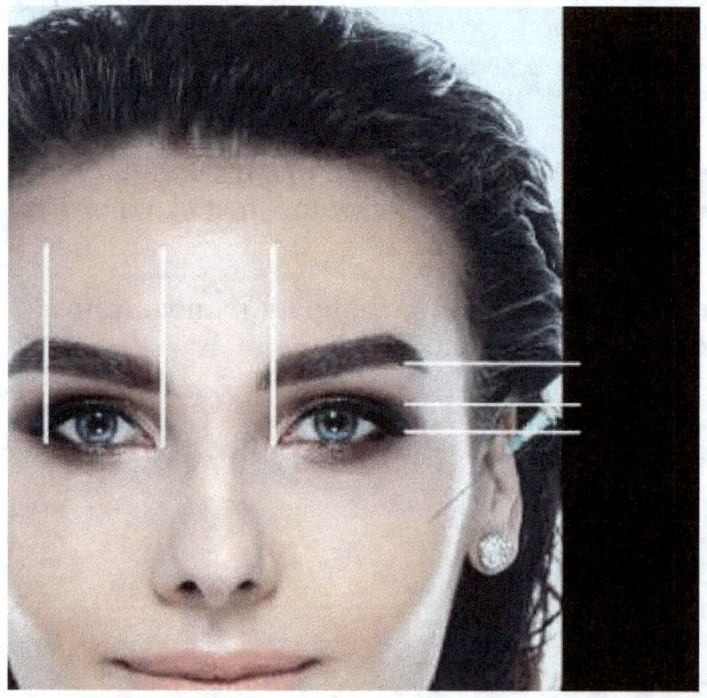

Using the proper color of contouring products, you can create the illusion of perfect eyes for a wide-set, close-set, droopy, deep-set, and bulging.

*Use a lighter color to bring out the lid and a darker shade to set that area back.

Eyebrows

Eyebrows play an important ole non-verbal communication, divert rain or sweat, soak up beads of sweat, and lastly, the bone and hair help to protect the soft part of the eyeball. Most important linear structure.

- Just with the brows, a client can change age with how they look.

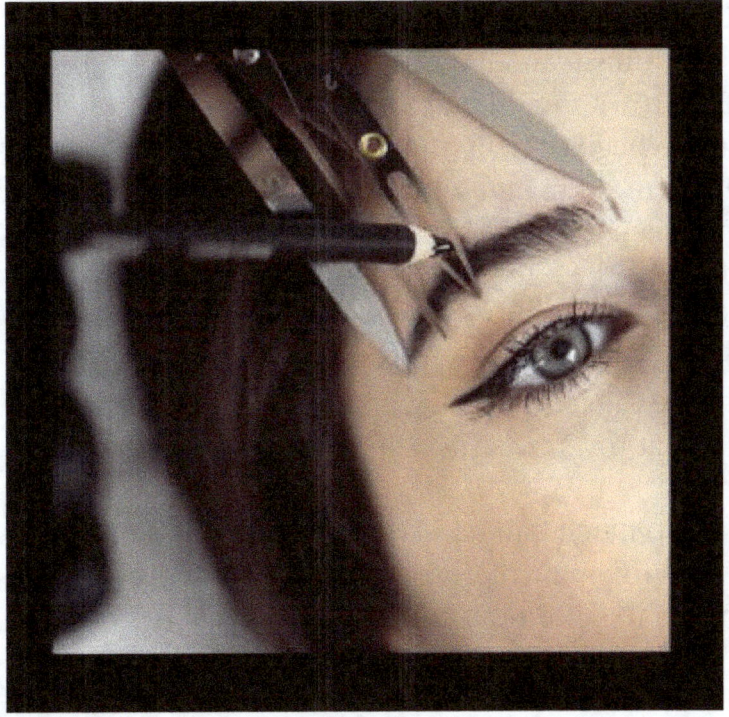

Perfect brows are spaced a specific way. Using an orangewood stick,

- line up from the inside of your nose to the inside of your eye... your brow should start in line with the stick.

- For the highest part of the brow, looking forward, line up from the inside of your nose to the middle of your pupil... your brow should highest in line with the stick.
- End of your brow, line up from the inside of your nose to the outside of your eye... your brow should end in line with the stick.

Tweezing the eyebrows

- Use a brow pencil to mark where the brow should start, finish, and have the arch.
- Eyebrows should taper from thick to thin (thickest at the beginning by the nose)
- Hold the skin taut with one hand by stretching it between the thumb and index finger
- Tweeze the hairs with the other hand in the direction of hair growth.
- Brush the hairs up with a brow brush, allowing you to see the base of the hair, and to remove the hairs in neat rows, creating the shape of the desired brow.
- *if too much hair is missing, use a brow pencil to fill in tiny hair-like strokes the look. Use a brow brush to soften the color and allow a more natural look.
- Or get them micro-bladed (the hair will eventually stop growing on the brows, so be careful not to pull too much hair) Women who pluck every day or wax their brows have poor structure and never get a shape (wait a week or two in between)
- Try never tweeze above the brow. When you get older the brows will fall, and you will not be able to pluck higher.

- Refer to waxing for information on how to wax the brows.
- Tattooed brows are always one color, no shadow of hair and light pops out.
- Botox makes you have one look always

ARE YOU READY TO PLAY?

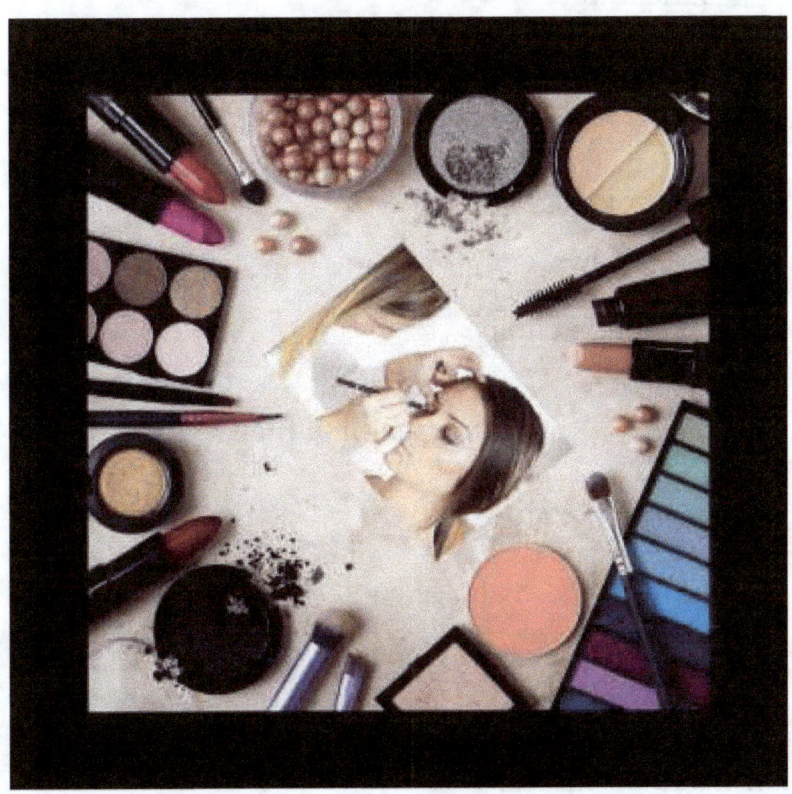

You are only as good as your canvas.

*A person's skin needs great skincare to have their make-up look good.

Quick Procedure:

1. Color of skin
2. Drape client (hair back in a pony if the hair is not styled)
3. Cleanser
4. Clarifier (toner)
5. Moisturizer
6. Eye serum or gel
7. Concealer & Counter Shading
8. Foundation
9. Blush
10. Eyes
11. Lips

1) What Color to Use?

Check the color of your client's skin

A) For foundation choice
<u>Skin coloring</u>

Cool — If their palm of their hand is - red, pink, or purple

-wrist blue

Warm — Palm of hand - orange, yellow

-wrist green

B) For make-up choice:

I. Should they wear warm or cool colors
II. What color of clothing will they be wearing?

C) What color are their Eyes?

    Cool — Dark rim and can see from the side angle

    Warm — Everyone else

    Porcelain color of skin use neutral eyes

D) What color is their Hair?
    Warm — Hint of red

You can use colored material to find out what color looks best

    Cool - Silver material

    Warm - Gold material

E) What is the clients color (skin and eyes)
    Warm skin = warm eyes = use warm make-up

    Cool skin = warm eyes = use neutral eyes

    Cool skin = cool eyes = use cool make-up

*You may choose to match make-up with the color of clothing.

Day Time Make-Up Procedure

1) Choose your colors

2) Drape client

> Cover the client with a towel over their clothes. Put their hair back with a headband, ponytail, or use your hand to move their hair out of the way.

3) Cleanser

> Excess surface cells look silver and flaky
>
> Healthy skin has a shine.
>
> Burning means take off- some people 30 seconds and some 1 ½ minutes...some products work to stimulate the skin and will cause a burning sensation.

    A. Put into the palm of your hand
    B. Wipe both hands together
    C. Holding the back of your hand on the client's forehead
    D. Wipe over half of their face (over eyelids) Forehead, nose, chin to cheeks -1x
    E. (Have client touch their face after each step, face should feel soft, clean, and smooth)
    F. Get the rest of the product off your hand and on to their forehead.
    G. Wipe on the other side of their face
    H. Remove-With 1st wet round sponge (yellow), wring out... Fold in half remove the cleanser, half of the face first, sideways motion, forehead down to chin.

I. Flip the sponge over and remove the cleanser from the other half of their face.
J. Have the client feel face

4) Clarifier/Toner

> A) To mist the face, start at the side of their face and then go over the face.
> B) Sponge face (swipe)

5) Moisturizer

> C) Put onto the back of your hand
> D) Put on the sponge from your hand
> E) Dab on cheeks, nose, chin, and forehead

6) Eye serum

> F) Eye gel
> G) Using Ring finger, tap under the brow and under eyes

7) Concealer

Wipe the brush on a tissue after use.

1.
- Red- green
- Orange- turquoise – standing in a pool, everyone looks good.
- Gold/yellow- blue
- Yellow/green- violet
- (Using complementary color will balance/ neutralize it. Look at their wrist for true color)
- Can blend colors to create the ideal color for your complexion.

-Yellow beige or Medium concealer – To diminish bluish shadows and moderate skin blemishes; covers pimples, pores, red blemishes

-Mint (green) - covers <u>red</u> only (nose, blemishes, rosacea, couprose on cheeks)

-Lilac – gives your complexion a healthy glow, use on your nose, chin, and forehead.

2. Counter Shading - Ivory or Light concealer - (brings things forward/closer) covers scars indents and dark circles. (can be used over dark or green)
    E on the picture)

    a. Corner of the eye to their hair
    b. Blend down & over
    c. Inside eye (if eyes are close-set)
    d. Nose if it has a dent(s)
    (tell the client they might want to wax excess hair on the sides)

3. Counter Shading - Dark Beige or Dark contour – shape and define
    A on the picture)

    a. Ear to chin dot (One side at a time so does not dry)
    b. Draw line with sponge pull down into chin (make it not seen)
    B on the picture)

    - Draw line at the ear (Knob of the ear)
    - Dab blend down swooshing towards the nose (ear to nose and back)

C on the picture)

- Wide nose - Blot sides with pad
(no extra concealer just with pad already used)

D on the picture)

- Hairline
- Chin line blot with pad

8) Foundation

    H) Put foundation onto inside of wrist
    I) Pat onto sponge (white sponge)
    J) 1st swipe away from the hairline
    K) Swipe across the eyelids (nose out)
    L) Look up – dab under the eye, then on top of the lid.
    M) Can swipe gently under the lid.
    N) Turn sponge to long side
    O) Dab over the face, all over to remove excess
    P) Pull foundation into hair line and ears
    Q) First make sure foundation is dry with touching use the back of the hand to cheek
    R) Powder in top of lid (1/4 tsp)
    S) Dip kabuti brush in and tap off
    T) Do swirls all over face from nose outwards. (helps dry up oil.)

9) Blush

    U) under the cheek bone (on dark contour line)
    V) ear to two fingers from their nose
    W) brush back & forth 2-3x, then up and down.

10) Eyes

- X) brow shape
- Y) brow powder where it is thin or no hair (may need tattoos or grow in hair)
- Z) 1a. light seashell inner eye lid 1/3 sponge brush
- AA) 2a. dark mud lid, outer eye lid (fluff brush)
- BB) 3a. liner pencil and powder (smoke look) side, then increase & lash line
- CC) 4a. eye shadow
- DD) Mascara – the bottom lashes and then the top lash (store mascara upside down)

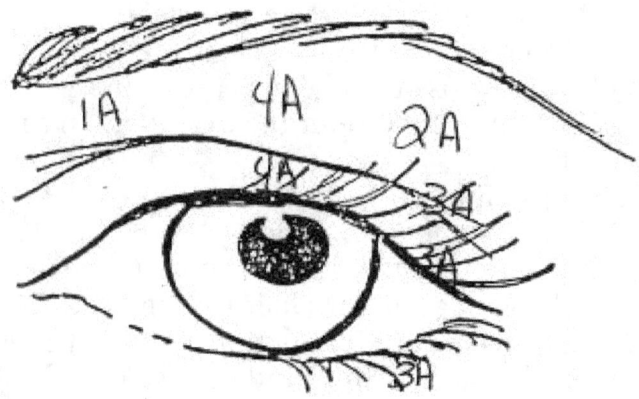

11) Lips

- EE) Liner (sharpen before and after)
- FF) Brush lipstick on
- GG) Vitamin E gloss, put all over or just in the middle of the lips

Extra Suggestions:

- Take before and after pictures of your clients
- Do not let your client watch you unless they are paying you for a <u>lesson</u>
- Product should feel cool on the skin
- Have client smell what you are putting on them
- Work from the side of the client (if you are right-handed... client's right side.)
- Kleenex –spray with vilex to clean your brushes
- The triangle sponge needs to be prepped (hydrate and moisturize) before you apply on the face
- Practitioner remove all jewelry /rings for cleansing
- Never <u>touch</u> clients with your fingertips or hands
- Use Q-tips to scratch face if needed, give to the client so they can use if need be.
- Lighting should be natural lighting, clear bulbs halogen
- Discourage a client from looking in a review mirror of a car (it is not their true look or color)
- Store mascara upside down
- For photos, do your hair and clothes first... Make up is put on last.
- Best brushes are goat's hair and sable (horsetail)

Natural facelift tips:

- Stimulate the muscles in the face, circulation - rush of blood and lymph.
- Skin becomes nourished and oxygenated & moisturized from the inside out.
- When there is more circulation the body produces more collagen
- Collagen gives the skin more tightness and elasticity.

Client Form

Copy or create your own version of this next page.

You can write what you used, and color what you used on the face (using what you used) in the appropriate area.

Date: _____ Client: _____ Signature: _____
Address: _____ Phone # _____
Practitioner: _____

Day Make-up ___ or Evening Make-up ___
Cover up
Concealer   _____
Foundation color _____
Powder
Shadow Base   _____
Shadow Crease   _____
Shadow Lid   _____
Liner   _____
Brows   _____
Cheeks   _____
Lip contour   _____
Lip color   _____
Lip gloss   _____
Finishing touches _____

Eyelash & Eyebrow Tinting

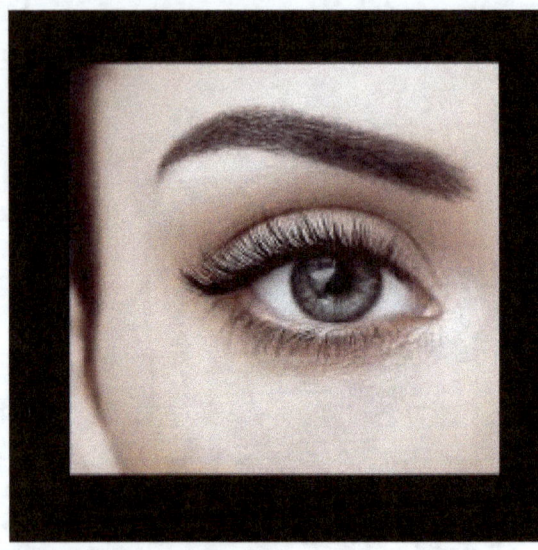

Creates the look of longer and darker eyelashes (not thicker), and darker eyebrows (can cover up grey hair). It is like hair dye for the lashes and brows.

Products needed:
- Cape or towels
- Cotton pads
- Developer Tint (appropriate color)
- Garbage Container
- Gibson Towel
- Make-up remover
- Paper Lower Lid Protector
- Q-Tips
- Rubbing Alcohol
- Saline Solution
- Scissors
- Tiny Dampen Dish
- Vaseline
- Water Dish

Last about one to six weeks (everyone is different).

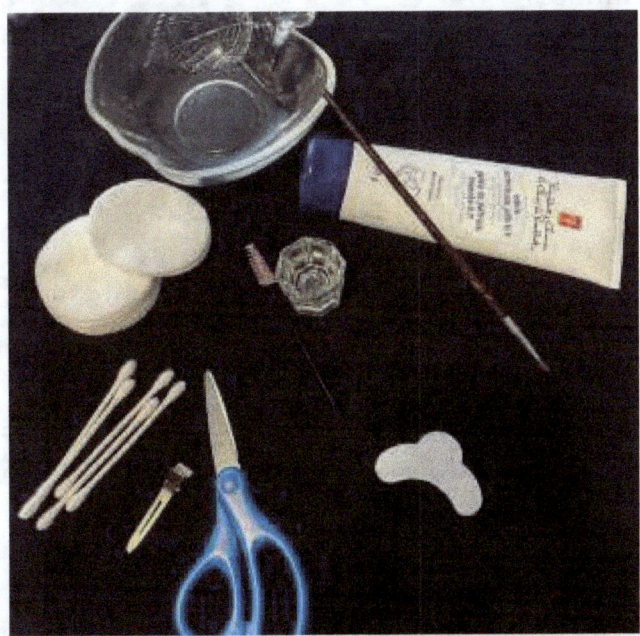

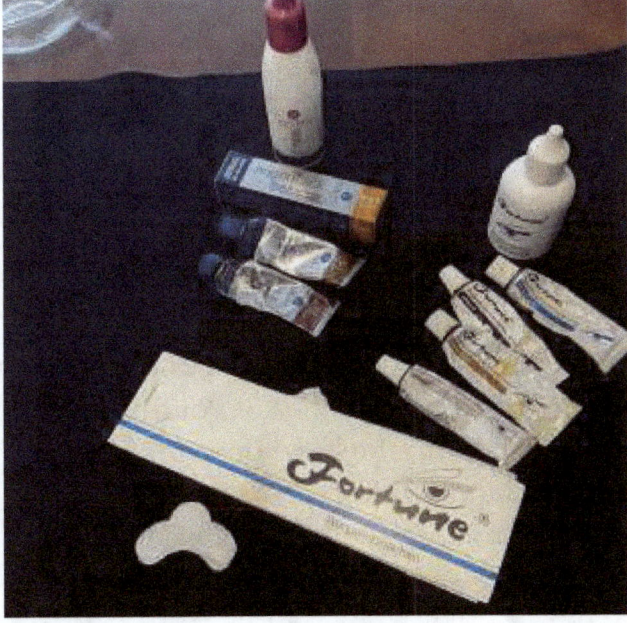

Shown here is two products that I like to use.

Lash Tint Procedure:
Time: 30 - 45 minutes

1. Set up your station.
2. Pre-cut the lower lid protectors to fit under the lashes of the client's eyes.
3. Sanitize small dampen dish & applicator.
4. Seat the client & drape the client's entire clothing (I have them lie on a massage table or in a lazy boy chair).
5. Prepare the tint. ½" to ¾" of dye (tube) and 8-10 drops of the developer (liquid). READ and follow your product instructions!!!
6. Remove any mascara.
7. Ask the client to look up, cut, and fit the paper eye protectors.
8. Apply the under eye protective cream (Vaseline) & place the paper protectors.
9. Ask the client to gently close their eyes.
10. Using the lash brush, sweep a small amount of tint on the underside of the lashes.
11. Lay the tint on the lashes thickly, causing the top lashes to adhere to the bottom lashes.
12. Using a magnifying glass, apply the tint to the base of the top lashes.
13. Allow the tint to remain on the lashes for 7 to 10 minutes (follow the directions of your product).
14. Dip a cotton pad into the bowl of water
15. Squeeze out and remove excess water
16. Tell the client to keep their eyes closed that you are applying the wet pad to remove the product now

17. Repeat a few times
18. Prepare Q-tips by barely moistening one side of the Q-tips.
19. Remove any remaining tint using a barely moistened Q-tip in a downward sweeping motion. Follow this with a dry Q-tip. Dispose of each Q-tip after one wipe. You may need up to 20 Q-tips for each eye before all the excess tint is removed.
20. At this point, ask the client to keep their eyes closed and that I am going to give them a damp Q-tip so that they can wipe clean any remaining product from their eyes.
21. Give the client as many Q-tips as needed to remove the product. They can open their eyes and get any product left in the corners.

*If at any time the client's eyes feel irritated, thoroughly rinse their eyes with the saline solution until any irritation is removed.

The Vaseline should have protected the skin from the tint, but if any tint is on the skin, remove it immediately after applying the tint. If doing brows, I use a dry Q-tip or two to shape the tint to the size I want around the brow

Brow Tint Procedure:
Time: 20 - 30 minutes
   (Both lash and brow, 30 - 45 minutes)

1. Set up your station.
2. Sanitize dampen dish & applicator.
3. Seat the client & drape the client's entire clothing.
4. Prepare the tint. Mix the tint to a slightly moister consistency than the lash tint mixture. ½" to ¾" of dye (tube) and 8-10 drops of the developer (liquid).
5. Remove any brow make-up.
6. Ask the client to close their eyes and apply the protective cream ½" around the row (Vaseline).
7. Using a swooping motion, apply the tint back and forth over the brow hairs (Brown shades only) try not to get on the skin.
8. Allow the tint to remain on the lashes for 1 to 10 minutes.
9. Remove the tint, in the direction of the hair growth, with a couple of dry cotton pads.
10. Immediately follow with a few barely moistened a cotton pad.
11. If any tint is on the skin, remove it with skin bleach. Then rinse off with cool water.

*If applying on both, lash and brows, apply the product on the eyelashes first then on the brows. Remove the product from the brows first, then the lashes.

*If at any time the client's eyes feel irritated, thoroughly rinse their eyes with the saline solution until all the irritation is removed.

The Vaseline should have protected the skin from the tint, but if any tint is on the skin, remove it immediately after applying the tint. I use a dry Q-tip or two to shape the tint to the size I want around the brow.

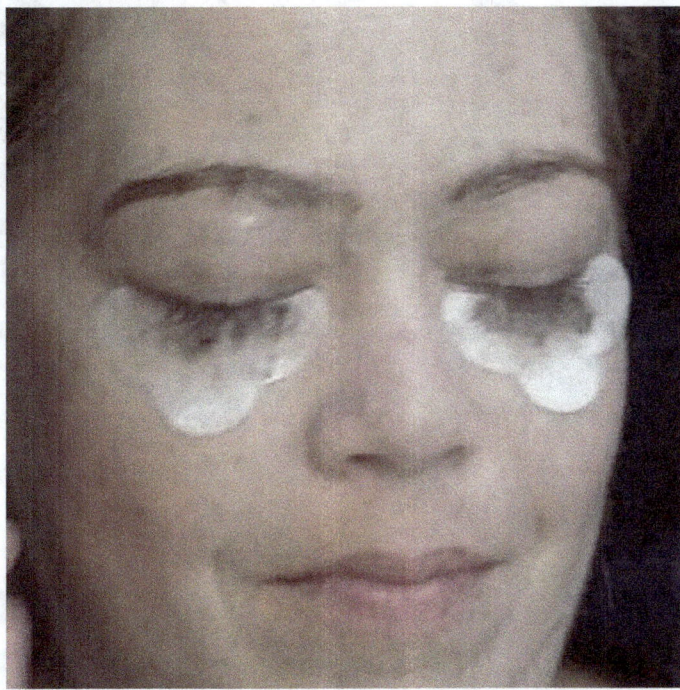

The color will always look different than it will be once you wipe off the product from the lashes and brows.

Waxing

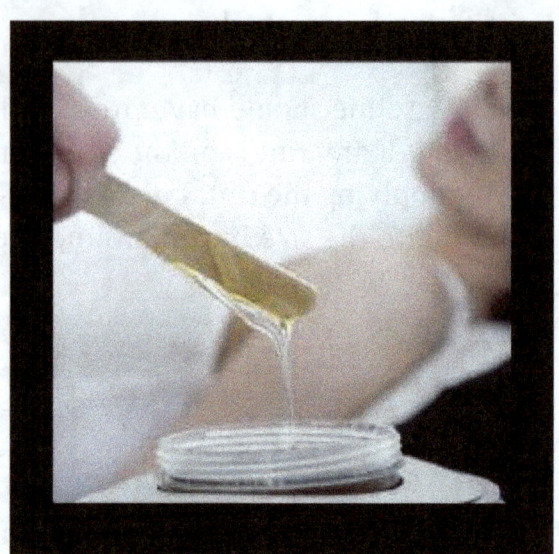

Trichology
Trichology is the study of hair, its structure, and its disorders.

Hair starts to develop when a fetus is 4-6 months old.

Location of hair on the body in percentile
- 50%   on head
- 16%   the body
- 15%   Auxilia (underarm, upper extremities)
- 14%   lower extremities
- 5 %   eyelashes and eyebrows

Hair also known as keratin is composed of 6 elements-
- S-   Sulfur
- H-   Hydrogen
- O-   Oxygen
- P-   Phosphorus
- C-   Carbon
- N-   Nitrogen

Definitions:
Papilla-

    Is the Mother reproduction organ of the hair. It receives the blood and is rich in nerve supply. It is the only part of a hair follicle that is alive.

Pilo Sebaceous-

    Unit- Includes the arrector pili muscle, hair follicle, and sebaceous gland.

Hair Follicle-

    The pocket that holds the shaft in the skin. It is a tube like shape.

Hair Shaft-

    The hair above and below the skin. The shaft is comprised of the cuticle, the cortex, and the medulla.

Bulb-

    The swollen extremity of the hair root which forms the lower part of the root.

Arrector Pili Muscle-

    A small tube-like muscle connected to the hair follicle. Fear and cold will contract this muscle. There are 2 areas of the body that do not have this muscle- the brows and the lashes.

Cuticle-

> The outer layer of the hair. A transparent layer of horn-like or scale-like shapes or plates of overlapping protective cells.

Cortex-

> The inner layer of fibrous cells fixed to each other, which gives the hair strength and elasticity.

Medulla-

> Also known as the Marrow or Inner Pith of the hair shaft. It may not always be there and /or it may contain air pockets.

Three Stages of Hair Growth

Composed of:

1) Anagen –

> A stage of like and action when the follicle grows down and the hair shaft grows up.

2) Catagen –

> The papilla follicle rises upward and pushes to the surface of the skin. Follicular degeneration occurs, and the hair falls out. The follicle breaks down if not in stage three.

3) Telogen –

> The resulting stage, though, if stimulation of the papilla occurs, re-growth can occur.

*** **IMPORTANT to know**... hair grows in threes. Meaning that if your client comes in and you do a waxing treatment, right after you pull the hair out or even the next day or two, new hair appears.

The only way to have no hair for six weeks is to have the hair removed every two weeks for three sessions, and then the hair will be removed approximately every six weeks.

Three Appendages to hair

- Hair Follicle
- Arrector Pili Muscle
- Sebaceous Gland

Hair color is determined by four things

- Genetics
- Melanin

Texture-

> The degree of coarseness or fineness of the hair is determined by genetics and whether the medulla is present.

Elasticity-

> The ability of hair to stretch and return to its original form without Breaking. Normal hair dry can be stretched to a 5th of its normal length Wet 40-50% of its length

Terminal Hair-

> Thicker, pigmented hair that grows on areas of the body after puberty

Lanugo Hair- Baby hair.
> It lacks oil glands, can be stimulated to turn into terminal Hair. Its function is to allow for temperature regulation.

Supercillia – Eyebrows.
> These do not have Erector Pilli muscles. The main function of eyelashes and eyebrows is for protection.

Epilation-
> Removal of hair from the follicle. Includes- electrolysis, waxing, plucking, and tweezing.

Depilatories –
> Temporary removal of hair.
>> Physical – soft and hard waxing – hair must be 1/8 – ¼" long)
>>
>> Chemical – Cremes (Neet, Nair)

Keratin-
> The primary component of skin cells found in two forms:
>> Hard keratin – fingernails
>>
>> Soft Keratin – skin & hair

SHOCK

Shock is the state of inadequate *perfusion* of the cells. *Perfusion* is the flow of blood to and from the body's cells. As blood flows, it carries life-giving oxygen and nutrients and carries waste away from the cells. The ultimate result of inadequate perfusion of each cell will be that it has too little oxygen and too much acid.

This will cause a series of changes:
- Cell function stops
- Cell dies
- Tissue dies
- Organ dies
- Body dies.

The fundamental problem in shock, regardless of causes, is a marked reduction in blood flow through the tissues.

Shock has many causes, including heart attack, sepsis (Meaning the presence of pathogenic organisms or their toxins in the blood or tissues), and physical trauma to the body. Trauma may be defined as any event or situation which causes physical distress and disruption. Trauma may include vehicular accidents, a fall from a height, or a sudden change in the body's functioning or homeostasis.

Homeostasis *(n)* is the ability or tendency of an organism or cell to maintain internal equilibrium by adjusting to its physiological process.

Everyone is unique in their tolerance to pain and change in the environment and situation. What for you or I may be a little "ouch" may be perceived by another person's body as a traumatic event. There is no reliable way to predict what a client's pain response will be.

The signs of shock are:
- Cool, pale, clammy skin
- Pallor in color
- Altered behavior
- Mental confusion
- Increased heart rate

In extreme cases:
- Poor capillary refill in fingertips
- Absent radial pulse
- Increased respiratory rate (panting)

Pallor and clamminess of skin are a result of the body diverting blood from the body's extremities to the vital organs; it is a life-preserving device for the body.

It is important to keep the client warm and calm. A client in shock will exhibit signs of distress; this is an unfamiliar and uncomfortable feeling for them. A client may feel embarrassment at their situation and may make statements such as "what a sissy" or "This is silly of me," "I can handle this." No one likes to admit that they are feeling less than "O.K." Especially when they have just had their leg, underarm, or bikini line waxed.

A client may become argumentative, they want the attention off themselves and they would really like to get away. It is important to keep yourself calm.
Ask Questions.

- Has the client eaten today? (Hypoglycemia)
- Is the client Diabetic, and have they taken their insulin properly? (Diabetic shock)
- Does the client have any known allergies (Anaphylactic shock)?
- Is the client using any other medications which may cause these side effects?

A client in extreme shock or distress is never to be allowed to leave the spa unattended or to operate a motor vehicle. Shock may progress quickly, and if unresolved, the results may be death.

A client in shock may complain of extreme thirst. However, water or liquids should never be given. The lips may be moistened instead while awaiting medical aid. Keep a record of the events leading up to the episode and the progression of the client's condition and notify a first aid attendant of the situation immediately.

The client may complain of feeling Dizzy, Woozy, and Shaky. A client who feels they are unable to stand on their own is to be encouraged to be seated in a chair with arms for support and covered for warmth Their feet should be elevated. **(* A client who must lie down must be transported to medical attention).** A client who is panting or feels like they have a "weight" on their chest will be reluctant to lie down and be encouraged to sit "up" in a reclining chair or supported by pillows or other bolsters. A client in respiratory distress is to be transported immediately to medical aid via ambulance.

A <u>pregnant woman</u> who exhibits signs of shock must be transported <u>immediately</u> to hospital, via ambulance.

It is always better to over-caution than to under-react.

WAXING PROCEDURE

- Contra-indicated if the client is on her menstrual (the skin is extra sensitive, and the procedure can be very painful).

SUPPLIES:

Wax Warmer	Powder
Wax	Baby Oil
Waxing Strips	Soothing Lotion
Examining Paper	Compresses
Tongue Depressors	Paper Towels
Cotton Pads	Tweezers
2 Large Towels	2 Small Plates
Rubbing Alcohol	

STATION SET UP:
- Plug in the wax pot.
- Clean the bed and cover it with the examining paper (like they use in a doctor's office).
- Place a clean towel on the pillow.
- Set up your supplies on a fresh piece of examining paper. Allow the paper to hang over the edges of the trolley or table.
- Place the baby oil on a small plate or in a pump.
- Have the wax warmer close to the edge of the table.
- Arrange the remaining supplies in the order in which they will be used.

PROCEDURE:
1. Have the client change into appropriate waxing garment (disposable underwear) or remove garments of the area that is going to be waxed.
2. Prepare the client's skin by lightly dusting it with baby powder.
3. The underarm area will need to be wiped with alcohol to remove any deodorant.
4. For the bikini line, the underwear will need to be protected with some paper towel or tissue.
5. Apply the thinnest amount of wax possible in the direction of hair growth.
6. Firmly apply the cotton strip in this same direction, rub your hand over the strip a couple of times (make sure the wax has stuck to the cotton strip).
7. Remove the strip in the opposite direction of the hair growth, using a low and straight back motion (do not create a large angle between the client's skin and the cotton strip when you remove it).
8. Pat or slap this area of skin in order to confuse/dull the pain receptors (I call it giving love to the area).
9. Wax the entire "front" area before you turn your client over to wax the "back" area.
10. Repeat these steps when waxing the "back" area on your client.
11. Apply baby oil to the entire waxed area.
12. Remove the oil with a very warm compress.
13. This serves to remove any residual wax.

14. If the underarm or bikini area becomes irritated, apply the soothing lotion. I love 'Azulene' skin-calming oil.

An allergic reaction may occur due to the wax. This is commonly expressed as tiny red papules. Assure your client that this is a common/mild reaction that will disappear within 2 – 4 hours.

If **<u>ANY SWELLING</u>** occurs, apply cold compresses immediately.

Body Polish/Scrub

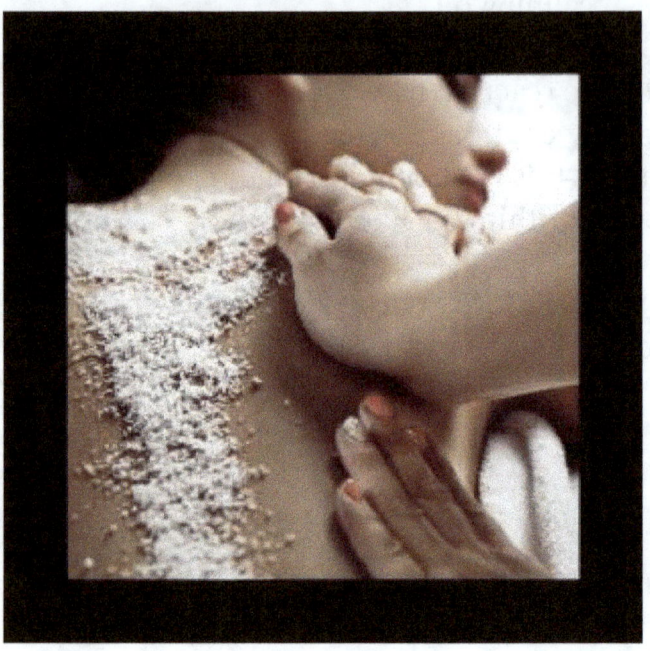

Procedure:
Time: 30 -45 minutes for a full body

1. Prepare the room for the client (create the mood)

2. Choose products; spa brand, sugar, oatmeal, walnut, salt, or Epsom salt scrub

3. Have client lie face down and pull the sheet over top of them.

4. Move the sheet to show the back of one leg. Apply the product onto the leg.

5. Lightly, start massaging the product on the leg

for a short period of time (2-3x effleurages).

6. Remove the product with hot towels, recover the body with the sheet.

7. Move the sheet to show the back of the other leg. Repeat last procedure.

8. Move the sheet to show their back. Repeat the similar procedure.

9. Cover the client and turn them over.

10. Move the sheet to show the front of one leg. Repeat the procedure.

11. Move the sheet to show the front of the other leg. Repeat the procedure.

12. For a woman client, towel and cover the breast area and reveal their stomach. Repeat the procedure.

13. Move the sheet to show one arm. Repeat the procedure.

14. Move the sheet to show the other arm. Repeat the procedure.

15. If the client would like you to do their face. If using salt, be very careful of the eyes. Sugar would be better to use.

16. You can have the client go and wash in a shower (if available) and come back for a full body massage, face massage, and scalp massage to finish. If not remove the product very well before massaging.

17. Gently awake your client if they have fallen asleep, telling them to get up slowly... help

them if they need it.

18. Meet them outside the room or at the front desk, have a glass of water ready for them.

Bronzing

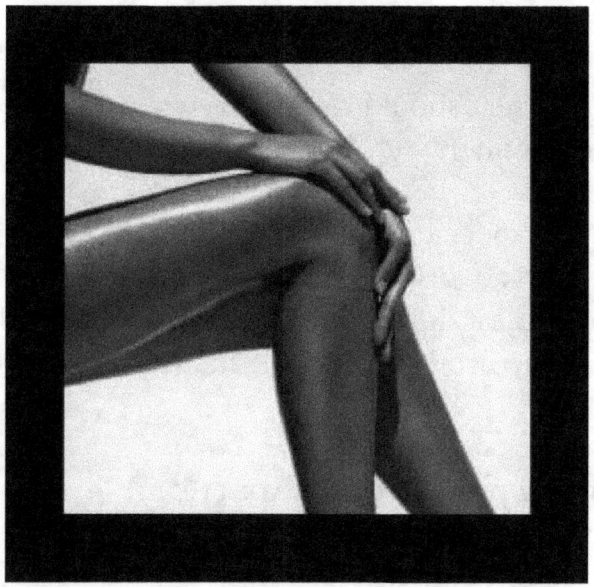

Best to be performed in conjunction with a body polish.

With the increase of sun damage to the skin, people are receiving an awesome tan without the UV issue. Many models, actors, grads, brides, and people going to fancy parties, love to have the look of bronzed skin.

Use a product that is an instant tan, not one that changes color within an hour. Some products leave an orange hue to the skin, test your product on yourself first before using it one a client.

There are many shades of color that you can purchase. I suggest having a few options for your clients (their own skin color will make a difference in the outcome). My favorite brand is 'So Bronze Professional Sunless Tanning, tinted self-tanning body lotion.' They also sell a bronzing mist.

The tanning effect should last about two to five days but can wash off sooner.

*If doing for a special occasion, have the client try it out a couple week in advance, so they know what to expect. I would also suggest doing the day before the special occasion, so the product does not stain any good clothing.

You will need:
- Tanning product (moose or cream)
- Plastic gloves
- Tissue like Kleenex
- Unscented lotion

Procedure:
Time: 30 -45 minutes for a full body
1. Have the client wear a bathing suit that they do not care about getting stained, or they can be nude or give them disposable underwear.
2. Have the client stand on a towel
3. Put on the gloves
4. Place a small amount of tanning solution in the palm of your hand
5. Mix a small amount of lotion in with it (the lotion allows a little more time and an even blend)

6. Use the tissue to blend and remove excess product
7. If doing the full body, start on one leg (do the foot of that leg last)
8. DO NOT repeat applying the product over the same spot (creates a darker area)
9. Apply to all areas the client wants tanned (face last)

Clean up
- If you spill any product INSTANTLY wipe it up
- Throw all tissue in a bag to place in the trash
- Remove your gloves and throw into the bag
- Use soap and water to wash your hands

Back Treatments

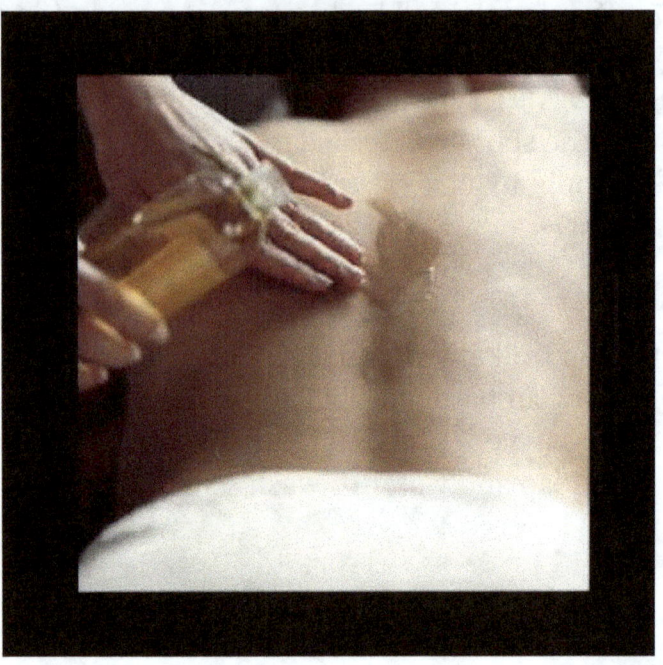

A back treatment is similar to a facial, but for the back. The back is cleansed, exfoliated, masked, and steamed to draw out and eliminate toxins and dead skin. A massage is given at the end to relieve aches, pain, and to relieve stress.

This type of treatment will help to
- Cleanse
- Moisturize
- Treat oily skin
- Treat acne prone skin

You can add paraffin just before the massage, for a deep healing effect. You can brush it on and let it sit for five to twenty minutes, then remove and perform the massage. Paraffin creates a warm deep penetrating heat, which softens the tissue, relaxes the muscles, and has been sued in therapeutic practices for arthritic conditions.

Procedure:
Time: 30 – 60 minutes

1. Prepare the room for the client (create the mood)
2. Choose the products (sensitive, normal, acne, mature skin, etc.)
3. Apply **cleanser**
4. Work in the cleanser, effleurage movements 3-4x
5. **Remove** with hot towels
6. Apply **toner**
7. Apply **mask**
8. Keep the client warm and covered while you wait (do a hand massage) 5-20 minutes
9. **Remove** mask
10. Apply **toner**
11. **? Paraffin** (optional)
12. **Massage**
13. Gently awake your client if they fell asleep
14. Ask if they need help to turn over or to get off the table.
15. Meet them outside the room or at the front desk, have a small glass of water ready for them.

Body Wraps

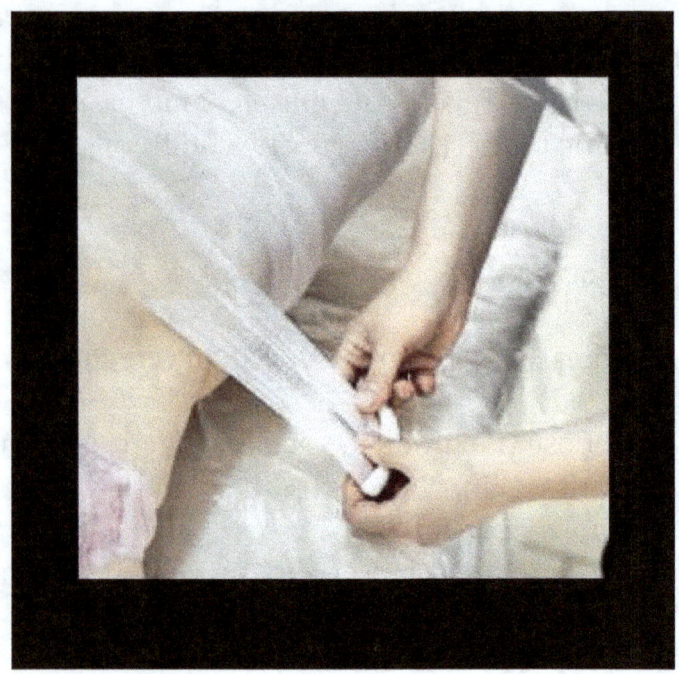

Contra-indications: If the client has
- high blood pressure,
- heart problems,
- or other medical conditions, such as high-heat situations
- or is pregnant

... then this technique may be harmful. Be sure to have the client consult their doctor before this procedure.
THEN DO NOT DO THIS TREATMENT

A SMOOTH, FIRM, HEALTHY FIGURE REQUIRES:

- Exercise to tone muscles.
- Proper diet, to regulate caloric intake.
- Plus... Detoxification to flush out stored wastes.

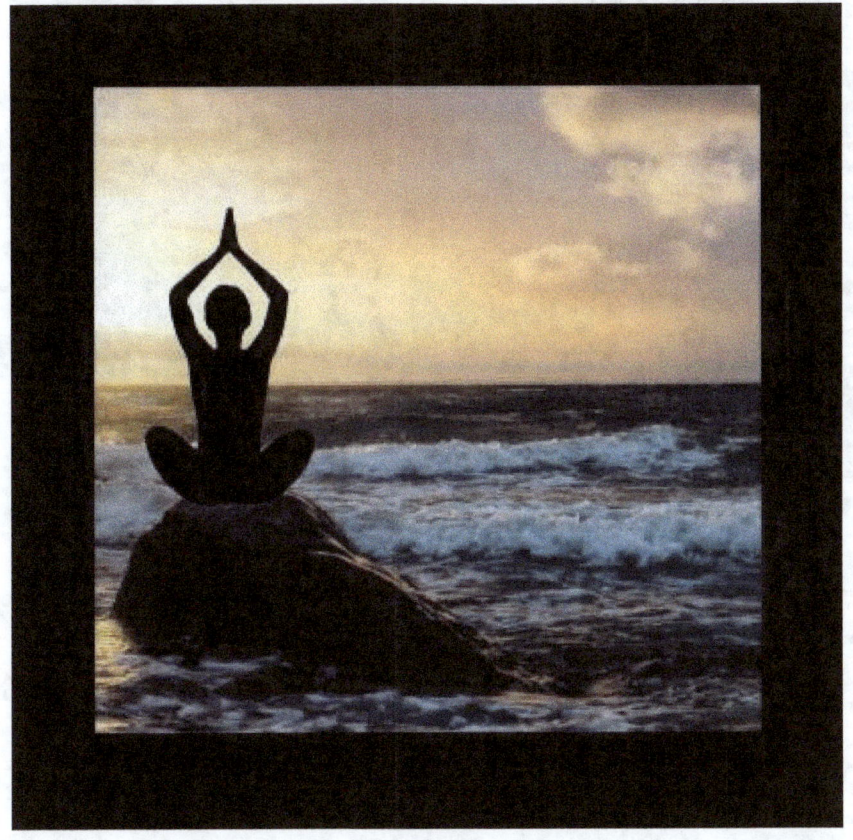

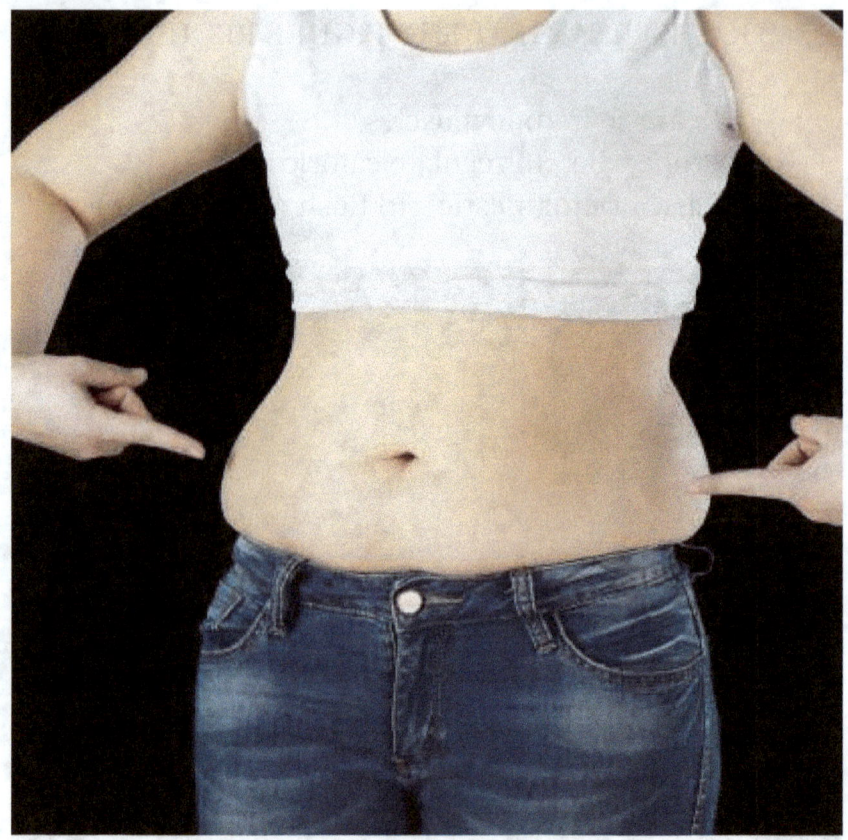

Bulges and heaviness from the...
- waist up is usually associated with overeating (Excluding medical problems).
- waist down is due to toxins and fluids stored in the connective tissue.

ANALYSIS AT A GLANCE
Description of correctable figure problems
and other conditions

CONDITIONS	CHARACTERISTICS	LOOKS	FEELS
1. Cellulite	Saddlebags	Starts at panty line, ends at mid-thigh - Lumpy	Bumpy
2. Water Retention	Flick Test: Surface skin will ripple	When depressed leaves white mark	Puffy
3. Thick ankles	No Taper	Whitish color & Bruising	Thick Hard
4. Lack of tone	Loose skin	Saggy	Not-resilient Loose –Soft
5. Thick upper arms	Hard bulging protrusion towards back of the arm	Blotchy Color	Rough surface Solid
6. Flabby upper inner arms	Loose & saggy skin	Loose	Separated
7. De-hydration	Crinkled	Look Dry	Dry
8. Sports Injury	Muscle Stiffness	Puffy	Warm

*Special Note:
SOME PROBLEMS CAN HAVE MANY ROOTS...
- FOR EXAMPLE, a **protruding stomach** can be:

1. POOR POSTURE - Improving the posture is still the fastest way to improve the entire figure
2. LACK OF MUSCLE TONE - Weak supporting muscles can allow the organs to fall forward.
3. ABDOMINAL BLOATING - The characteristics of this type is that the abdominal protrusion can come and go from day-to-day - can be caused by gases or fluid retention.
4. CONSTIPATION - Characteristics are the abdomen protrudes and feels hard to the touch - often involves overuse of laxatives.

ANALYSIS OF CORRECTABLE FIGURE CONDITIONS

All figure problems fall into three different categories:

1. EXCESS FAT CAUSED BY: **Excessive caloric intake for frame and activity level**-- Begins on the upper part of the body. Characteristics: - Heavy upper arms - Thickening on the back - Breast enlarging - Double chin - Fat pockets on the back of hips (upper buttocks) - Abdomen and waist thickening
2. LOCALIZED FAT POCKETS CAUSED BY: - **Stored wastes and toxins** - Hormonal imbalances - Chemicals and additives in foods that overload the body's ability to eliminate excess wastes. Characteristics: - Cellulite saddlebags - Thick ankles - Fatty pockets on the inner knee - Fluid retention anywhere on the body i.e. legs, back, abdomen, hands, feet or under eyes
3. LACK OF TONE OR FIRMNESS CAUSED BY: **Lack of exercise** Characteristics: Flabbiness, loose skin that has a sagging appearance occurring on: - Inner thighs - Inner upper arms - Buttocks (causing ripples on back of thighs) - Abdomen - Breasts

THREE TYPES OF FIGURE PROBLEMS

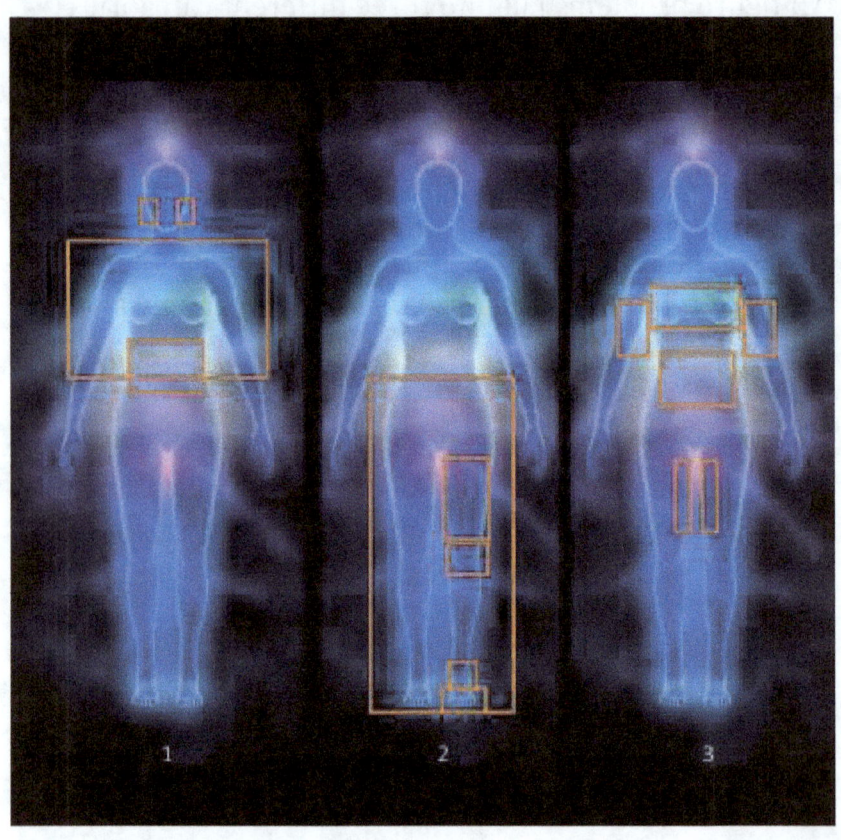

1. Excess Calorie Intake
2. Stored Toxins
3. Lack of Tone (Need for More Exercise)

Placement of packs, wraps, and body masks

Localized Packs

Recipe Choices

- Detox
- Re-mineralizing
- Placement – Full body wrap (different product, different places)
- Product
    - Detox: Mud or clay
    - Re-mineralizing: Seaweed or Herbs

Compression Wraps

Recipe Choices

- Detox
- Placement – Arms & Legs or Contour Wrap
- Detox Product – Mud or clay

Total Body Masks

Recipe Choices

- Detox or Re-mineralizing
- Placement – Full body wrap
- Product (one or the other product)
    - Detox: Mud or clay
    - Re-mineralizing: Seaweed or Herbs

TYPES OF FAT CHARACTERISTICS & REMEDIES

To be successful in treating skin and figure problems, the esthetician of this decade will rely much more on their analytical abilities. Just as a physician's competency is judged by their diagnostic skills, so will the esthetician be judged by their analytical skills.

The following outline explains the different types of fatty tissue, its characteristics, its appearance, and the appropriate treatment methods.

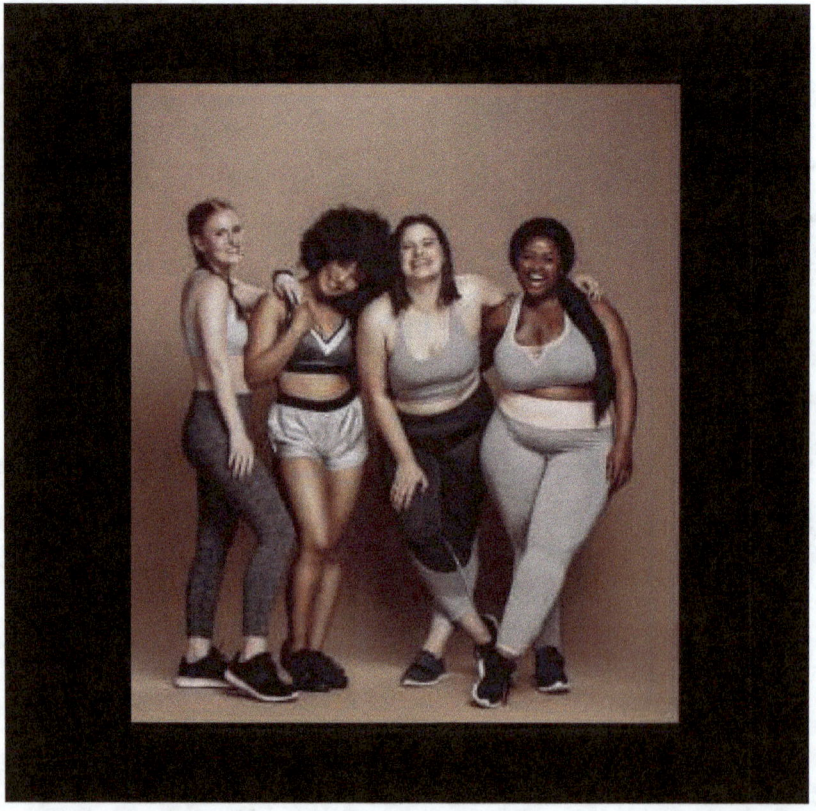

TYPE I: HORMONAL FAT

CHARACTERISTICS: When firmly stroked you will feel, (deep inside the tissue), soft lumps about the size of marbles.

LOCATION: Accumulates mostly on the outer thigh and inner knee.

REMEDIES: Seaweed compression wraps to unlock trapped toxins. Calcium magnesium capsules three times daily to help control fluid retention. Seaweed baths at home for maintenance and to prevent future build-up.

NOTE: To treat this particular condition, it is not necessary to use heat. Detoxification should take place through stimulation of the lymphatic system.......not through perspiration. Results are immediate after the very first treatment when using seaweeds.

BEST TREATMENTS CHOICES FOR: Hormonal Fat (Example: Cellulite)
- SEAWEED TREATMENTS,
- THERMAL HEAT

TYPE II: SOLID DENSE FAT

CHARACTERISTICS: Firm fat with yellow coloration of the skin in the fatty area.

LOCATION: Begins and accumulates in the upper part of the body i.e. back, arms, chest, neck, and mid-torso.

REMEDIES: Thermal heat treatments with seaweed to help breakdown solid, dense fat. Proper diet with a nutritional consultation. Seaweed capsules three times daily with meals to help improve metabolism.

NOTE: If you do not have a nutritional consultant on staff, it is a good idea to compile a list of recommended tapes and books.

BEST TREATMENTS CHOICES FOR: Solid, dense fat, mostly on the upper body
- SEAWEED TREATMENTS,
- THERMAL HEAT,
- EXERCISE,
- DIETING

TYPE III: FLUID FILLED TISSUES

CHARACTERISTICS: Soft with no yellow coloration. The surface has a ripple effect when flicked.

LOCATION: Appears over all fleshy areas of the body.

REMEDIES: Internal calcium/magnesium capsules three times daily to act as a diuretic. Total seaweed detox body mask to remove the excess fluid from the tissue and stimulate the lymph for the final elimination of excess fluids from the body.

NOTE: First treatment brings immediate results.

BEST TREATMENTS CHOICES FOR: Fluid Filled Tissues. (Example: Occurs more frequently 2 weeks before menstruation).
- SEAWEED TREATMENTS,
- THERMAL HEAT
- AND LOW SALT DIET

TYPE IV: SOLIDLY INFILTRATED FAT

CHARACTERISTICS: Tissues feel hard and solid. The skin has an obvious whitish appearance. Lack of visible vessels through the skin in that area. When depressed leaves while mark.

LOCATION: Usually, affects calves, ankles, and feet.

REMEDIES: Body brushing, in the direction of the heart, to stimulate lymph flow. Seaweed baths and localized seaweed detox packs to unlock trapped fluids in skin tissue. Cal-meg capsules to prevent future fluid build-up.

NOTE: Never use deep tissue massage because it forces the fluids back into the tissue.

BEST TREATMENTS CHOICES FOR: Solidly Infiltrated Fat. Example Thick ankles.
- SEAWFED TREATMENTS,
- LOW-SALT DIET

TYPE V: FLABBY FAT

CHARACTERISTICS: Loose, sagging appearance to the skin - total lack of tone.

LOCATION: Whole body: face, neck, breasts, buttocks, thighs, upper arms, etc.

REMEDIES: Seaweed mineralization baths at home to hydrate and elasticize tissue. Seaweed capsules three times daily to re-mineralize the tissue. Electric muscle toning machine. Exercise.

NOTE: This can appear in any or all areas of the body. Home maintenance must include exercise to tone muscles.

BEST TREATMENTS CHOICES FOR: Flabby Fat. (Example inner thighs and sagging upper arms).
- SEAWEED TREATMENTS,
- TONING MACHINE,
- EXERCISE

God's Gift to the World
ALGAE

Dictionary Definition: 'chlorophylls sea life, without roots or blood vessels. Grows in seawater, freshwater and even from moist air.'

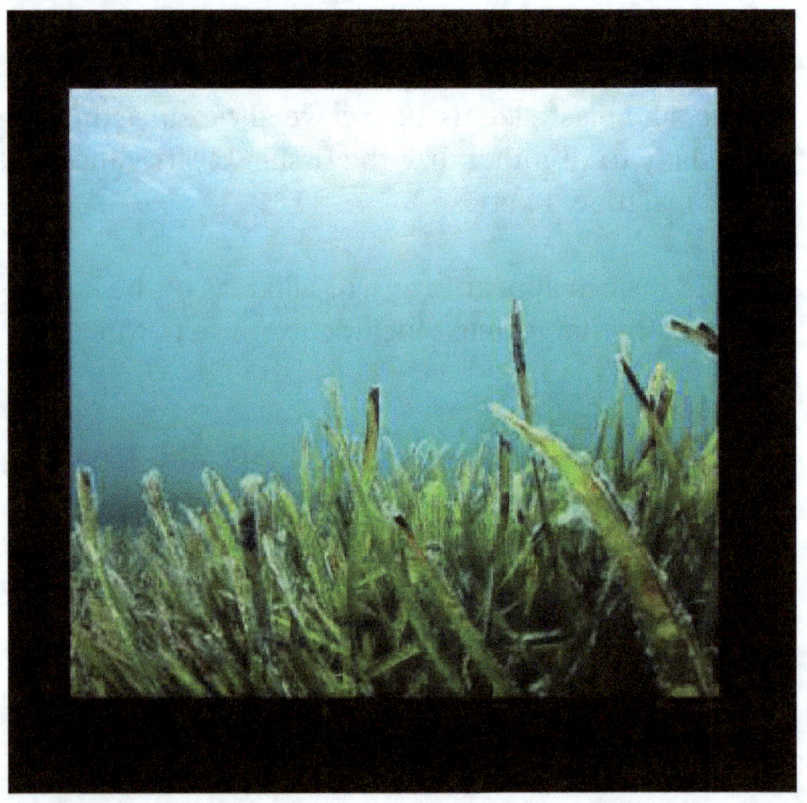

*Closest cell structure to the Human cell, are skin eats it up like food.

Generalities:
Throughout the ages, we have always known algae as a sea plant that enriches the soil. From the recent studies of professor Augier, U.E.R. researching on sea life sciences, we now know more about the real properties and active principles of Algae's, along with the specific and important role they play in the growth, maturity, caliber and preservation of plants and their by-products (unknown up to now, was the discovery of female phytohormones belonging to the algae family).

Marine algae have exceptional properties and, if kept fresh up to the time of use, will retain 95% of their properties. This is due to their being collected and treated during their prime and in their natural environment. Algae treated in this way are rich in 60 oligo-elements and act directly and favorably on cell growth as well as promoting the regulation of cell division.

There are surprising results from the use of algotherapy in the field of cosmetology including:

- Prevention of hair loss,
- acne treatment,
- blotches on the face,
- heavy legs,
- development and firming of the breasts,
- cellulitis treatment,
- slimming,
- rejuvenation of the skin etc.

Skin treated with certain varieties of algae has a much younger and healthier life span. Some of these elements allow better absorption and a maximum binding of phosphor and calcium. This is done through the chlorophyllous exchange. Due to this exchange, the skin develops a strong resistance to infections and sensitivities.

General points on Algae:
Marine algae are as profuse as land flora- today, we list as many as 865 varieties, and over 700 of those species are on the coast of B.C.

Algae are a life form belonging to the vegetable family; formed of identical cells, they neither have sap nor root systems. They have an osmosis interchange, cell to cell- and grow through mineral elements found in seawater.

Reproduction occurs through the spores on an annual basis. Building occurs during autumn and winter, maturing between February and May (Northern Hemisphere)

Conditions of a good algae crop:
1. Harvested in spring while in full biological activity
2. Deep sea sites where strong tidal currents knead and oxygenate the algae.

Scientists could extract penicillin from algae
- 500 g of algae is equal to a synthesis of 10,000 L of seawater
- Algae are richer than thermal and mineral waters
- They contain all the basic nutrients
- They are bactericidal
- They are antibiotic (acrylic acid)
- It is not said "life comes from the sea" The much-used word Thalassotherapy (seawater therapy) comes from Greek: "Thalassa", the sea; "Therapy", to cure
- 72% of the oxygen we breathe is produced by Algae.

People who include sea-foods in their diets are less prone to certain ailments and diseases than others, simply because seawater possesses all the minerals and elements required for good health.

Marine plants grow in an environment rich in minerals, which they absorb and retain, they affect the transition of mineral to an animal. The minerals travel through the organism of those who feed on and are dependent on Algae. Everything on land, in oceans, and in the human body exists as a consequence of this fine balance.

Algae in the diet:

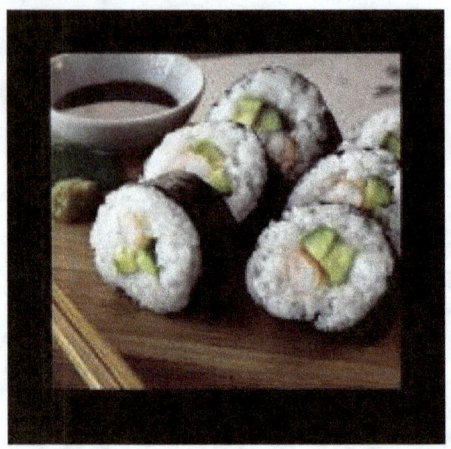

In Japan, algae constitute more than 25% of the national diet and are prepared in many different ways.

In Ireland, Denmark, and other maritime countries, one can find algae at the dinner table. Dr. Quintou has established beyond question that the liquid obtained by the boiling of algae, has the same substance as the lymphatic liquid in the human body. The same oligo-elements found in algae are also found in human metabolism. Algae play an essential and irreplaceable role in the basic function of the metabolism:

- *Sodium Chloride* - provides a balance of acid-base
- *Magnesium* - favoring organism defenses, activates cellular functions.
- *Calcium* – anti-allergy, regulates the neuro-vegetative system
- *Potassium* - stimulates diuresis, important heart action
- *Iodine* - acts on the thyroid, blood vessels, aging, tiredness
- *Copper, Zinc, Manganese* - stimulates and rebalances the glands with internal secretion (endocranial system)

Composition of fresh Algaes
Macro Elements

Nitrogen	1.50%	Sulphur	2.50%
Phosphor	0.50%	Magnesium	4-6%
Potassium	3%	Calcium	2-3%

60 Oligo Elements

Iodine	2100	Stronium	50
Iron	1500	Aluminum	75
Manganese	260	Barium	15
Boron	70	Titanium	12
Cobalt	2	Arsenic	8
Copper	12	Silver	1
Zinc	40	Gold	2
Bromine	3	Chromium	1
Nickel	7	Pewter	80
Fluorin	30 (Teeth concentration)		

Amino Acids

Cystine	Glutamic	Arginine	Lysine	Tryptophane
Proline	Orniathine	Aspartic	Methionine	Phenilalamine

Vitamins Lipo and Hydrosolubles

A	E	D	C
	(Antihaemmohagie)	(Used in Pharmacy)	
PP	B1, B, B12	B	K

Phytohormone

Natural vegetal hormones of growth (female phytohormone)			
	Abscissines (anti-ageing)		
Auxines	Cytokinines	Laminarines	

CHEMICAL COMPOSITION AND EFFECTS OF BROWN ALGAE ON THE SKIN TISSUE AND BODY.

AMINO ACIDS
- Works on the reconstruction of weakened.
    - arginine
    - aspartic
    - cystine
    - glutamic
    - lysine
    - methionine
    - ornithine
    - phenylamine
    - proline
    - tryptophan

MACRO ELEMENTS

- Acts on cellular activity, cellular exchanges, and re-minerals the skin.
    - azote
    - calcium
    - magnesium
    - phosphorus
    - potassium
    - sulfur

PHYIDHORMONES
- Plant hormones that promote healthy growth and act as a gentle stimulant to rebalance hormonal imbalances:
    - abscisins
    - alginates
    - auxins
    - chlorophyll
    - cytokinins
    - gibberellins
    - laminarians

TRACE ELEMENTS
- Stimulates fast biological reactions in the tissues.
    - aluminum
    - arsenic
    - barium
    - bromide
    - boron
    - chromium
    - cobalt silver
    - copper
    - fluoride
    - gold
    - iodine
    - iron
    - manganese
    - nickel
    - strontium
    - tin
    - titanium
    - zinc

SEAWEEDS:
- ASSIMILATE into the tissues and create cellular exchanges, to cleanse and rebalance the body's deficiency.
- PENETRATE the skin because of their likeness to the human tissues and fluids.

VITAMINS
- Helps compensate for the deficiency.
- Fat and water-soluble

Depending on the seaweed...
- A
- B1
- B2
- B12
- C
- D
- E
- K
- PP

Mummy Wrap Procedure

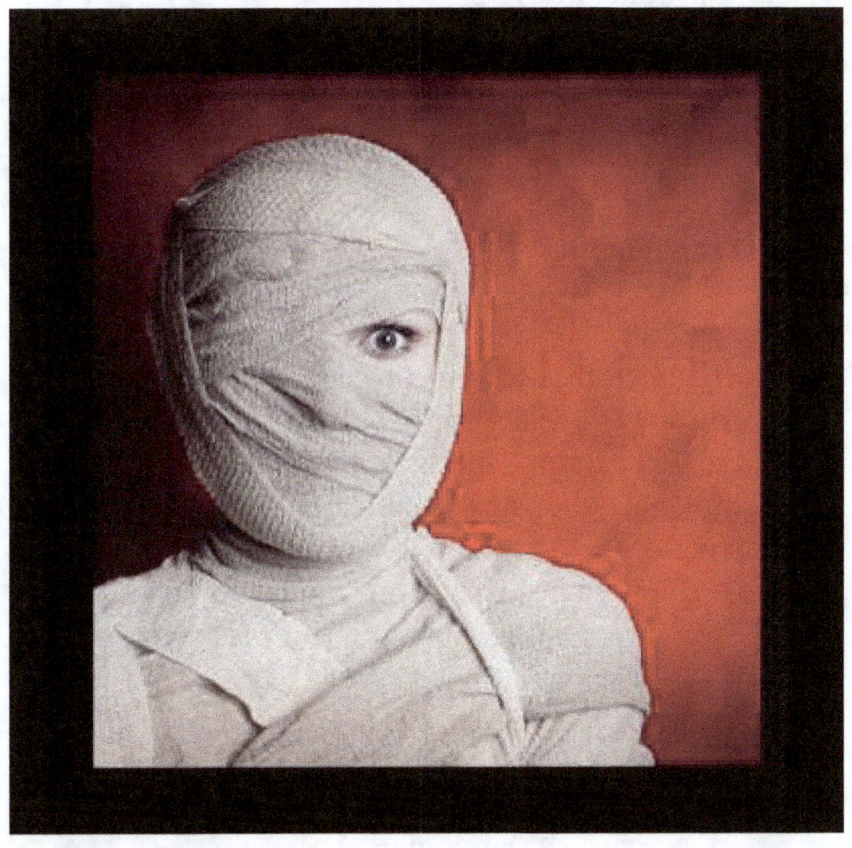

Okay, we do not ever cover the mouth and nose... but we do wrap...

I am more interested in you learning the technique of wrapping then the product you use (each Spa will carry a different product line)
- Some use a sheet process instead of the 'mummy' technique.
- Some use elastic or plastic wraps instead of cotton wraps

Body Wrap Supplies

You can buy already made linen body wraps or buy the fabric (cheesecloth, wide cotton gauze Linen, or loose-weave cotton) and make your own.
- Cut 10 of them 4 inches wide x 9 feet long. (Some students cut up an old cotton sheet and use that to practice).
    o For a bigger person, you might need twelve.
    o Depending on your client's size, you will use:
        - 1– each calf
        - 2 · 1– each thigh
        - 2 · 1– hips
        - 1– abdomen
        - 1– breast
        - 1– shoulder
        - 1– each arm
- Products – Herbal, Mud, or Clay (depends what reason you are doing the wrap for).
- Massage Table
- Towels
- 2 Big bowls
- Crock Pot

Linen Body Wrap Set Up & Procedure

1. Make sure you have told her ahead of time that she will need to bring an extra pair of under clothing.
2. Soak body wraps (linens) in water first then add to crockpot (you will need ten to twelve)
3. Pour liquid solution over linens.
4. Prepare table: you will need insulated gloves, tongs, and stainless-steel bowl.
5. Layout a plastic suit (rain suit), so it is handy.
6. Have bed prepared as well
7. Have massage oil ready in a glass container or squeeze bottle.
8. Lay a large towel down on the floor for your client to stand on while you wrap her.
9. Greet your client and explain what she needs to do in the room. Get her to take off her clothes down to her underwear or swimsuit. Have her stand on the towel with a large towel wrapped around her for warmth.
10. Leave room for her to change. Knock before entering.
11. Begin wrapping from the top of the leg down to the ankles. Remember, if it is too hot for you to hold on to, it is too hot to put on them. Fan it to cool a bit first.
12. Wrap both legs.
13. Wrap the client's mid-section (hips and abdomen).
14. Put on the plastic pants.
15. Wrap the client's arms.
16. Wrap the client's breast and shoulder area.

17. Help the client get into the plastic jacket.
18. Help your client to lie down on the massage table.
19. Cover the client with the sheet and blanket.
20. Do a facial massage, hands, and or feet.
21. Remove the wrap after 20 minutes unless the client is uncomfortable than remove sooner.
22. Stand the client back up on to the towel.
23. Give the client a large towel to cover themselves with.
24. Have the client remove their under garments if wearing any, and then go back under the sheet and blanket (make sure to keep them warm).
25. Finish with a full body massage. ELD massage is best.

Massage Table Body Wrap Procedure:

1. Have herb, mud, or clay mixture made
2. Lay the plastic drop cloth over the massage table
3. Lay the silver emergency blanket over the drop cloth.
4. Lay the blanket over the silver one.
5. Dip and Soak the cotton sheet into the herbal mixture.
6. Wring out the hot cloth and...
7. Wrap the client and lie them on the massage table or place sheet on the massage table and have client lie down and then wrap them.
8. Wait about 10 - 20 minutes (you can give a head massage during this time).
9. When finished, tell the client not to bathe for 12 - 24 hours. They can get dressed and meet you at the reception desk.

Cellulite Body Wrap Session (Dry)

Cellulite is hardening tissue deposits due to ineffective circulation and elimination, not enough water, and hormonal issues.

Client needs to do a two-week internal cleanse and for ultimate success, a weight loss program for eight weeks.

Supplies:

- Plastic Circulatory Brush
- 2 Spatulas
- Vinyl gloves
- Plastic Blanket or Saran Wrap
- Silver Thermal Blanket
- Large Blanket (wool works best)
- 2 pillows
- 2 Large towels
- 2 Hand towels
- Flat Sheet
- Client needs a bathing suit or use disposable linen
- Optional -2 hot packs
- 30 drops Rosemary & Lemon Essential Oil
- Carrier Oil
- Cream
- Mud

Procedure:

Cover massage table with:

- blanket first
- thermal blanket
- sheet if not using a plastic blanket

1. Start with the client facing downwards. May use pillows if needed (stomach and under ankles).
2. Cover the client with a large towel.
3. Check where cellulite is on the leg.
4. Apply Essential Oil to upper leg (cellulite area)
5. Brush towards the heart (until the skin is Hyperemia – red) approx. 2 minutes
6. Apply cream and work in
    a. Effleurage
    b. Knead
    c. Roll the skin
    d. Squeeze together and roll
    e. Form a 'v' and knead
    f. Finish with a drain

Check with the client if the pressure is okay. The client should feel it but not major pain.

7. If you use a vibration machine (G5 or GX99), use now.
8. Do all sections of the body.
9. Can turn the client onto their back.
10. Apply ample amount of mud onto the cellulite area and wrap in plastic (remove air/seal by smoothing with hand)
11. Mummy the client by wrapping in a thermal and warm blanket.
12. Cover the top of their head with a towel.
13. Can apply hot packs.

14. Leave the mud on for 20 minutes.
15. Remove sections of mud individually with a spatula. (Can take the excess of mud and wipe on plastic). Remove remaining with DRY towel.
16. ELD Massage.

- They will have sessions 3x a week for 7 weeks (21 times).
- Then 1x every 6 weeks for 5 sessions.
- Then once or twice a year after that.

Home care:

1. In the shower - brush body.
2. Apply the cream in the morning (Rosemary and Lemon Essential oil mixture)
3. Mud bath every night.
4. Apply the cream in the evening. (Ylang Ylang and Lemon Essential oil mixture)

Mud Body Wrap
Supplies and Procedure

10 Bags of body wrap mud
A warmer that holds up to 30 bandages
30 Tensor bandages (if you also want to do contour wrap)
    – Prewash and dry, twice, to have the bandages work properly
Two big towels
4 little towels
2 bed sheets
Pillows
Raincoat and pants <u>or</u> thermal outfit
Big bowl

Mud - Heating up the mud in warmer:

1. ***Depending on what type of warmer you bought, you may need to put water in between the warmer and the metal container for the burner to stay wet. Read direction from the manufacture.
2. Pour <u>1 liter</u> of water of hot water into the container
3. To start the mud
    a. Pour 1 bag of mud into the water and stir until the mud is completely mixed into the water.
    b. Mix all the bags of mud into container (add a bit more water if need be).
    c. *(the mud left over after a client, can be kept on low heat for the next client).*
   When starting with a new client:
4. **All you have to do is pour 1 new bag of mud into the water and stir until the**

mud is completely mixed into the water.
5. Put <u>15 bandages</u> into the container
6. Pour enough hot water over top of the bandages to cover them.
7. Mix <u>half</u> of the new bag of mud onto the bandages.
8. Mixing mud and water over the bandages.
9. Put the remaining <u>15 bandages</u> onto of the other bandages and add enough water to cover the bandages, and now add the rest of the mud from the bag and mix.
10. No big chunks of mud should be left.
11. Remember to clean the mud away from around the warmer as the salt from the mud will rust any metal.
12. Heat the mud for one hour before starting with the client.
13. Check the bandages after 30 minutes and move the top bandages to the bottom in order for all the bandages to be heated up equally.
14. *The bandages should be hot but not too hot in order to apply to the skin.
15. Have the massage table set up before hand with sheets and blankets.

Procedure: (takes about 1 ½ to 2 hours)

1. Have the client fill out the contra-indications form.
2. Once they have completed all necessary documents, have the client undress and stand on the towel (*It is beneficial for the client to be completely naked in order for the most detoxification to come out of their body. If they are not comfortable,*

give them throw away underwear in order to not get their own clothing wet).
3. Using the tape measure, you will measure the client starting at their chin working all the way down to their ankles. Follow the form.
4. The client will continue to stand on the towel while you wrap them.

Start with their legs.
5. You will first begin with one of their legs. Wring out two bandages and place in the bowl, so no dripping happens.
    a. Make sure the bandages are not dripping of water!
    b. You will wrap inward and upward towards the heart. Start at the ankle and work your way up. You might need up to 3 bandages if the client is a bit bigger or taller in size.
6. To get the most benefit out of the wrap, you can use another bandage over the thigh area to tighten the areas after you have applied the flesh (first area) bandages. Repeat from just above the knee and slightly tighten the bandage as you pull upward and inward over the thigh.
7. Repeat the same procedure on the other leg (opposite direction).

Tummy and bum
8. You might need up to 2 bandages. Wrap just below the belly button to bottom of bum area.
9. You will need up to 6 bandages. Start from the thigh and wrap around one leg and then go to the opposite side of bum and lift and slightly tighten to firm up the bum area. Repeat on the other leg. And

keep repeating on opposite sides until all six bandages are used.

Waist

10. You might need up to 2 bandages. Wrap bandage from under breast area around to below belly button. (The client needs to breathe, so make sure tight but not too tight).

Breast

11. You might need up to 4 bandages. Wrap around the breast area (with breasts being lifted into a higher position). Can go over the shoulder.

Arms

12. You will need 1 bandage per arm. Start at the wrist and work to the underarm. You can go over the shoulder.

Shoulder/Breast area

13. You might need up to 2 bandages. From one side to the other with a bit of a lift to the breast area.

Head

14. You will need 1 bandage. (Not all clients are okay with this one, do not do if they do not like it) Wrap around the head and neck, lifting the chin area. Make sure they can breathe!

Suit

15. Put the suit on them and have them lie down on the massage table
    a. Put a pillow under their head and one under their knees.
    b. You can massage their feet and hands.
    c. You can place a blanket over them.
    d. Have them lie there 15 minutes to one hour (read directions from the mud package).

  e. If you leave the room, check in on them every 15 minutes.
16. Help them to stand back up and remove the suit
17. Start to remove the bandages (give them a large dry towel to keep warm!).
18. Let them dry off for 15 minutes before you re-measure them (When they are wet, they will be larger than when they are dry). They can lie back down on the table and cover up.
19. Once they are dry, you can re-measure all the areas.
20. They can get dressed now.
21. Figure out the difference of the measurements.
22. The client can book one session each week for 3 to 5 weeks, then once every six months, or for a special occasion.

NATURAL COSMETICS

Aloe Vera
Moisturizing used in skin creams. For injuries, burns, and skin problems. Healing abilities

Almond Bran
Use in facial scrubs and masks. Exfoliating Almond bran with water makes an excellent facial scrub. For dry skin use Almond Oil

Avocado Oil
Great source of Vitamin A, C, and E. Excellent healing qualities. Soothes eczema promotes regeneration of scarred skin. Treats scaly dried skin and scalp.

Arrowroot
Foot and body powder. Mix with essential oils to make body talc.

Beeswax
Beeswax derived from the honeycomb is naturally yellow. White beeswax bleached by air and sun may cause allergies. Beeswax is a natural emulsifying agent that makes creams and lotions smooth or hard.

Clay
Clay is the best mask that you can use on the skin. Clay clears the skin, stimulates circulation, and is anti-inflammatory. It draws out toxins, contains minerals, Green clay is suited for oily skin. *Mature skin does not usually need clay or mud masks.*

Cocoa Butter
Excellent moisturizer. Used to mate creams and lotions

Coconut Oil
Excellent source to be used in creams

Chamomile
Flower Use in facial masks, eye creams. Great for sensitive skin.

Dulse
High mineral content draws out impurities. Use in Thalassotherapy body wraps and herbal facial lifts.

Flower Waters
Flower waters are created when essential oils are obtained through the steam distillation process. These oils and water have a rejuvenating effect on the skin. Great to use as toners and body spritzer. Antiseptic, cooling and astringent

Glycerine
Colorless syrup used to bind, lubricate, or dilute cosmetic mixtures. Used in soap, moisturizing, dilute with flower water to make a body spritzer. 12

Honey
Used in preparations of creams, lotions, masks, and in the bath. Great for all skin types.

Jojoba Oil

Jojoba oil does not have color or smell, therefore, ideal for skincare. It is one of the best oils used for facial treatments. A faci1 oil made with jojoba and essential oils could have more properties than any expensive skin treatment. Excellent for facial massage.

Kelp Seaweed.

Emollient, rich in vitamins and minerals Used in Thalassotherapy body wraps, masks, and bath treatments.

Lemon Balm

Cleansing, antiseptic. Use in a facial steam.

Milk

Contains vitamins and protein. Use fresh whole milk in baths for sensitive skin. Add honey for dry skin and wheat germ for blemished skin. Use whole milk in masks instead of water.

Sweet Almond Oil

Is a high quality oil that absorbs well into the skin. Will help to absorb essential oils. Best carrier oil for the face (except jojoba). Sweet almond oil is derived from the ripe seeds or sweet almonds from the almond tree. Smoothes and maintains the skin. Yellowish in color and odorless. Wonderful for making skin-care oils and creams.

Vinegar

Apple cider vinegar is an inexpensive beauty aid that can be mixed with essential oils to rinse calcium remnants and soap residue from the hair. Vinegar is also helpful against dandruff. Added to the bath, it cleans greasy, blemished skin. Facial skin is particularly well cleansed by a mixture of vinegar, pure water, and a few drops of peppermint. Great for aftershave lotion.

Wheat Bran

This by-product of flour production is valued for its soothing, anti-inflammatory, and healing qualities. Bran contains vitamin B6, which is important to cell removal. Its main use is in skincare, baths, and masks. Wheat bran cleanses the skin and makes it soft.

Witch Hazel

Witch hazel is an alcoholic extract from the leaves & flowers. It is used in cosmetics because of its healing, toning, anti-inflammatory, and astringent qualities. Pure witch hazel is a great toner. Works well for mature, tired, sluggish, oily blemished, and infected skin. Great as an aftershave.

Yogurt

Yogurt contains lactic acid and can be used externally in masks and body wraps. Great as a moisturizer, but also works well for oily and blemished skin. Eating yogurt is the best natural way to care for the skin.

BODY WRAP RECIPES

Material needed:
- Your favorite herb or combination of herbs
- Cotton sheet and Plastic drop doth or shower curtain, or mummy wrap
- Silver emergency blanket
- Blanket
- 2 Big Bowls
- Massage Table

Herbal Body Wrap

- ✓ Fill a large sink or bucket with very hot water.
- ✓ Place chosen herbs in a pot and fill with water.
- ✓ Bring to a boil and simmer 15 minutes.
- ✓ Cover for 5 minutes.
- ✓ Scoop out as many herbs as possible.
- ✓ Soak linens.

Recipe for Relaxation Body Wrap

Material needed:
- 6 cups boiling water
- 3 cups fresh herbs:
- 1 cup chamomile chopped
- 1 cup valerian grated
- 1 cup lavender crushed
- ✓ Place herbs in a pot and fill with water.
- ✓ Bring to a boil and simmer 15 minutes.
- ✓ Cover for 5 minutes.
- ✓ Scoop out as many herbs as possible.
- ✓ Soak linens.

Spa Style Herbal Body Wrap
- 2 cup dried chamomile
- 1/2 cup dried rosemary
- 1/4 cup fresh mint or peppermint leaves
- ✓ Place herbs in a pot and fill with water.
- ✓ Bring to a boil and simmer 15 minutes.
- ✓ Cover for 5 minutes.
- ✓ Scoop out as many herbs as possible.
- ✓ Soak linens.

Castor Oil Wrap

Excellent for scar tissue and fibroids

- Soak a white cotton cloth in Castor Oil (cut cloth size of issue)
- Place the cloth on the area that has the issue
- Saran Wrap the area (all the way around so nothing moves or leaks out – Not too tight)
- Sleep with the wrap overnight
- Repeat each night for three days – if doing uterus fibroids, repeat until you are urinating oil

*Make sure what you are wearing and sleeping on is old, Castor oil can stain.

What Makes A Great Practitioner?

Personal and professional ethics within the spa
For a minute, let me give you a scenario and then tell me what you think:

You and a friend walk into a spa for a day of pampering. You pay for your appointment, and you sit and wait for the wonderful person who will pamper you for the rest of the day. Your name is called, and you look up to see a young woman (we will say) you first impression is her hair is a mess and looks at her lab coat it is covered in stains. You brush the thought off, and she takes you to your room, opening the door and saying, "Take off your clothes; I'll be back in a minute!" You are wondering what to keep on, which way to lie on the table, or do I get on the table now?

When she comes back, she barely gives you time to get on the table now and starts your facial already! As she leans over you, you smell cigarette smoke on her clothes and her breath.

The smell bothers you, but you continue because you have already paid for the session and want to feel good. All the while, the woman talks only about her life and the partying she did with her friends the night before. She never kept quiet the whole time!

The young woman rushes you through the service, making you feel rushed and in a whirlwind of stress from the moment you walked in the door.

Now, let us talk about how you would feel in this situation. Do you feel that this was a good value for the dollar you have spent? This is not only an insult to your client but to yourself as well as the spa in which you work. Your impression is what keeps you coming back, and sometimes, if your personality is wonderful, they will come back to see you even if your service was not one hundred percent.

In the spa industry, personality is everything. It is your personality that can calm a client if they are in for the first time or nervous about removing clothing for a massage. Your ability to make the client feel at ease and know that they can trust you is what will keep them coming back for more. The client will also give you a wonderful recommendation to friends and family members if she has a positive experience with you.

HYGIENE AND PROPER GROOMING:

<u>Appearance:</u>
Present a clean, neat, and attractive appearance. This does not mean you must look as if you are going to the ball, but if your hair is longer than shoulder length, have it pinned up or pulled back. Keeping your skin looking refreshed with a little bit of make-up, such as mascara, blush, and some lipstick. Even a little will go a long way towards making a great impression.

For men, keeping a clean-shaven beard or mustache neatly trimmed is a must.

- Daily bath or shower and the use of deodorant are essential.
- Hand bathes or shower daily.
- Because of client sensitivity issues, use no perfume or cologne.
- Always have extra deodorant in your purse, locker, or car (wherever you can get to it). Many services may cause you to stain, when the room gets warm, you may begin to perspire.
- Never trust that you are okay, always be prepared for the worst.

<u>Clothing and shoes</u>:
Whether you wear a uniform or your own clothing, it should be clean, neat, pressed, and properly fitted. Try to present a conservative, professional image rather than super-sexy or stylish.

I recommend a smock with shorter sleeves to wear over your clothing, a neutral colored top that does not show past the sleeves of your smock. There is always a possibility of splashing oil or other product on your clothing; in this way, you can take the liberty of protecting your wardrobe and looking professional at once.

If working with an Esthetician or in another professional office, a recommendation is a colored smock which offsets the color of the others in your office, making you look unique and recognizable. Always wear a nametag, telling others who you are.

- Estheticians usually wear white smocks
- Spa Practitioners usually wear black

Hands and Nails:
Hands should always be clean, nails trimmed, and well cared for. Nails should be clean, trimmed, and if polished, only light or clear nail polish used. Clients will judge your spa and your service based upon what your nails and hands look like. A mani-care client will observe your own hands and nails to draw clues as to what sort of service you are able to provide. And a massage client will appreciate your courtesy in not scratching their skin with long or jagged nails.

Fatigue:
Fatigue and tiredness resulting from work, exercise, mental effort, or the strain caused by hurry and worry tend to drain the body of its vitality. Therefore, an

adequate amount of sleep, not less than seven hours is necessary.

Thoughts and emotions:
Your thoughts and emotions influence your body's activities. An angry thought may cause the face to turn red and increase heart action. A thought may either stimulate or depress the functions of the body. Strong emotions influence the heart, arteries, and glands. Mental depression weakens the functions of the organs, thereby lowering the resistance of your body to disease.

A Healthy attitude:
The mind and body operate as a unit. A well-balanced condition of the body and mind result in good health. This enables you to perform all bodily functions normally. A healthy attitude can be cultivated through self-control. In place of worry and fear, the health-giving qualities of cheerfulness, courage, and hope should be encouraged. Outside interests and recreation relieve the strain and monotony of hard work.

Graciousness:
Learn to display pleasant emotions. A smile, greetings, a word of welcome, the willingness to assume the responsibilities of friendship, the ability to fit into new situations, and to meet new people with friendliness all are part of professionalism. A sincere smile sets the mood for warm human relations.

Politeness:
The root of politeness is the thoughtfulness of others. It includes the little things such as, "thank you" and "please," treating people with respect, exercising care of others' property, being tolerant and understanding other people's efforts and being considerate of those for whom you work.

Voice and conversation:
Tone of voice, conversational skills, and good language skills equal success. The use of proper grammar and intelligent conversation will serve well as a professional spa practitioner. Remember that success is not made within the salon alone but also depends on personal contacts, associations, and active participation in many social and business functions.

Good Ethics:
Ethical behavior is a simple, straightforward matter.
1) Be honest, but tactful, with all of your clients
2) Treat all clients fairly and with equal respect
3) Be dependable in all your dealings with clients, co-workers, and others
4) Take the initiative in solving problems for your clients and for your spa
5) Always practice the highest standards of professionalism.

Poor Ethics:
1. Questionable practices, extravagant claims, and unfulfilled promises violate the rules of ethical conduct. These acts make yourself, others

within your profession and your entire industry look bad.

Look at the list below; recognize examples of how you should be greeting your customer and how so many simple things can make your client recognize you as a professional.

1. Greet clients warmly and introduce yourself with a light, using a confident handshake
2. If they are aged, help them if they need it. A helpful arm will do as you walk them to your treatment area.
3. Take their jacket if they have not hung it up at the entrance
4. If this is the client's first time in your spa, fill out your client consultation. The client may be a repeat customer and have information on file, which you will go over quickly to make sure nothing has changed (Medications, pregnancies, or injuries).
5. Give adequate instruction as to what to do to prepare for their service, keep in mind this may be her first time receiving this kind of service.
6. Assure the client that you will step out and be back shortly, at which time you will knock on the door to let them know you are there. Do not enter until they say, "come in."
7. Enter quietly.
8. Keep your voice calm and reassuring at all times. Remind the client that this is 'their time.' They may choose to converse with you, or they may

choose to relax completely, and maybe even have a little nap.
9. Always be aware of your client's body language under your hands. You should be able to recognize if she or he is hurting or uncomfortable. Do not be afraid to ask how the pressure is, and if the client is comfortable.
10. If you are offering a service that requires conversation such as a manicure or pedicure, then talk but keep the conversation focused on the client. Let the client talk to you and keep your conversation neutral- weather, how they are feeling etc. Stay away from a conversation about your own life or family, unless it adds something to what the client is talking about.
11. When the service is complete, help the client get up. If lying down, give them a few minutes to become balanced and ask if they need assistance off the table. Let them know you will meet them in the reception area. Remind them to put their jewelry back on.
12. Remember, if you are sick with a cough to always wear a mask over your mouth. Sometimes a virus can come on at work, and you do not want to pass it along to your clients. Explain tactfully that you are coming down with something or have allergies and would like to use a mask. They will appreciate your attention to their wellbeing.
13. Always wash your hands before and after every client, and use a cream to soften your hands as

well. Keep your hands warm if possible and warm them before touching your client.
14. Remember to always prepare your room at least fifteen minutes before the appointment time and set up for one client at a time. This means lighting, music, product, towels sheets, and paperwork. Set your table to the proper height. You do not want to break contact with the client once established.
15. Always ground yourself before each service. You may not think a stressed-out client has any effect on you, but the truth is they do. You may absorb their stress. Take a few moments to breathe and center yourself before moving on.
16. You may tactfully mention another service your client may want or need. This is called up-selling, and it benefits yourself and your peers to learn to do it well.
17. Before your client leaves, book their next appointment. This is easy to do with facial, manicure, pedicure, massage, or waxing.
18. Be honest. Clients will appreciate your honesty much more than fantastic claims you and your spa could never live up to.

Always keep in mind that the service you would want will be the service your client will also want from you. If you enjoy certain things, most of the time, so will your clients. Being able to communicate well helps with up selling and re-booking.

Make sure you have had an experience with all the services your spa offers so that you know how to explain them to your client. It is easier to explain something if you have had the service and liked it as well.

Client Consultation

A client consultation is your method of record keeping. It enables you to save time by recording the results of your treatments, how many they have had; if they have purchased any products, if they liked the product. A client consultation record will also protect the practitioner from false or malicious claims made by clients.

This kind of record-keeping also enables you to cut set-up time down by quite a bit. By referring to the client record, you can see which products they have used and what comments were made. It is important to include medical history, medications, and allergies as well. Modern day cosmetics can cause allergic reactions or sensitivities for people sensitive to smells and to chemicals or additives put into a product.

The client consultation paper or card—most spas use one form or another. You can add or change this form for your own practice but always make sure the necessary elements are included.

- The client's name, address, and home phone number. If your client asks you why you want her number, simply explain that your spa does promotions throughout the year and that you call

your clients in person to tell them about it. It is also a nice way to send greetings over the holidays,
- Any information regarding medical treatments, medical history, and vitamin supplements they are taking, pregnancies, heart problems, etc.
- Notice any abnormalities of the skin. Do a personal consultation when you have them settled in the room before their service. This ensures privacy. You may ask the client to fill out general (name, address) information in the waiting room, but you will do the rest with her or simply wait and do everything at once.
- Make sure to record any allergies.
- Note any marks, bruises, or injuries.
- If your client is dieting, note her weight and age when they come in for record's sake.
- Ask if they were referred to your spa and how they heard of you. This helps you track which advertising is effective.

Your client consultation is your window into the client. It also helps with regular clients to remember their name, birth date, etc.

Keep track and always call your client by her first name or preferred title.

Bibliography

Many definitions are from Wikipedia, the free encyclopedia

Artwork is mostly from canva.com or my own photos

Brummet, Connie

    2000   Canadian Institute Of Natural Health & Healing, Day Spa & Esthetics Courses

Milady's Skin Carfe & Cosmetic Ingredients Dictionary, Natalia Michalun, www.delmar.com

The Beauty Bible, 2nd Edition, Paula Begoun

The Skin Type Solution, Leslie Baumann, M.D.

Salon Fundamentals, Student Manual

Associations:
Leading Spas of Canada
    https://www.leadingspasofcanada.com/

Beauty Council
    https://beautycouncil.ca/

For more information about Leading Spas of Canada and the Quality Assurance Program, contact:

    www.leadingspasofcanada.com

Trade Shows

    https://vancouver.spa-show.com/

    https://www.iecslasvegas.com/exhibit

Suppliers and Courses:

Look under Beauty Suppliers & Equipment.
*You will need a copy of your student ID card, or a certificate of graduation, or a business license to get in.

You can use saran wrap, real wraps or cut up an old sheet and use that in the wrap.

www.newdirectionsaromatics.com (check country)
www.goldenmoor.com
www.keyano.com   Keyano Aromatics
www.phyto5.us
www.casmara.us
www.saian.net
www.eminenceorganics.com/us
www.mbicanada.com
www.maccosmetics.ca
www.lisewatier.com/ca_en
www.footlogix.com
www.universalcontourwrap.com

Beauty Store
www.iconbc.com

Cosmo Prof/ Monarch Beauty
www. stores.cosmoprofbeauty.com

ESP salon sales
www.espsalonsales.com

West Coast Beauty Co.
www.west-coast-beauty.com

Modern Beauty Supplies
www.modernbeauty.com

West Coast Beauty
www.west-coast-beauty.com

Nail Techniques
www.nailtechniques.com

Also check at
London Drugs
Shoppers Drugmart
Grocery stores

Message From The Author

Even though I am taking a break from Mani's and Pedi's, and studying for my PH. D in Integrated Medicine, I cherish the knowledge I have learned.

I am so grateful I know how to help myself and my family look after their bodies... a little pampering now and again never hurt anyone; in fact, it has helped many people to de-stress. Which is a miracle all on its own.

I hope you have enjoyed the Secrets of a Healer Series, and I hope that you will take the time to learn what you need to gain health, wealth, and happiness.

Shift happens... Create magic!

Love and Light Constance

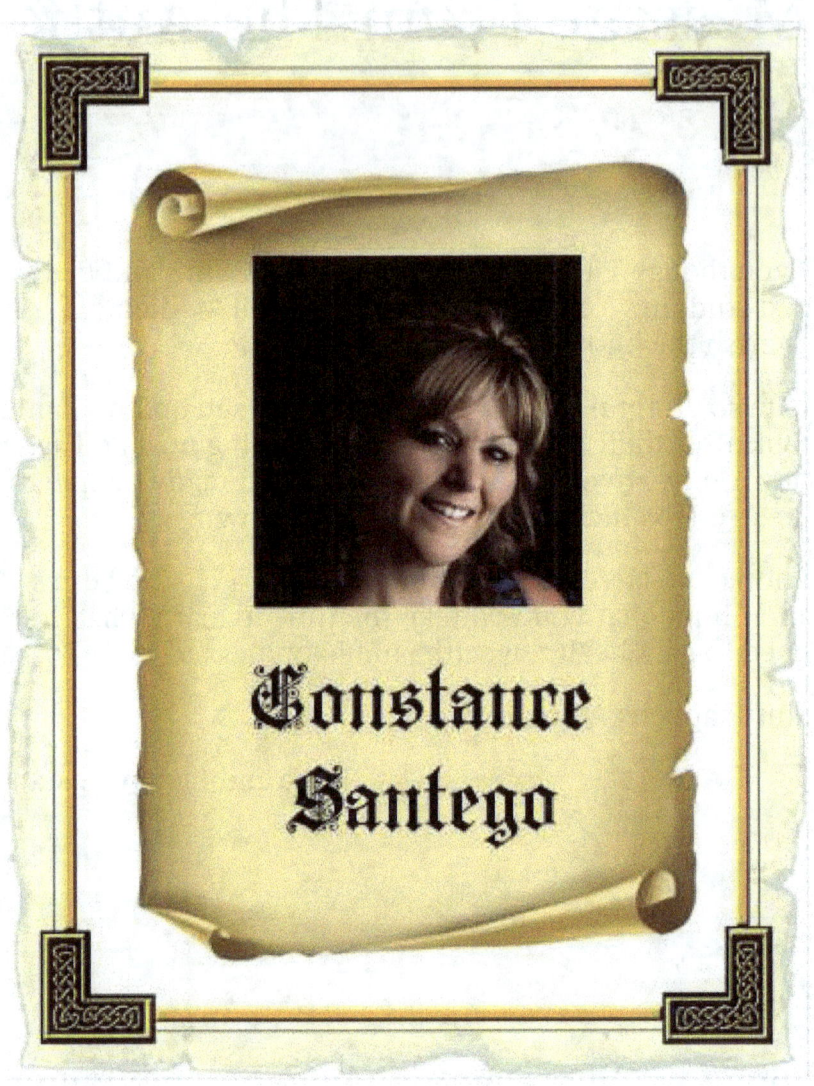

Shift happens...Create magic!
Dream BIGGER!

Constance Santego is an Author, Master Educator, Hypnotherapy Teacher, and Healer of the Holistic and Spiritual Arts. She is known for bridging the body, mind, and soul consciousness to create your dreams into reality.

Constance's background is in business, owning her first company at the age of twenty-seven until her back went out and she had to sell. Learning how to heal herself holistically, she gained many, many certificates and diplomas in spirituality and natural healing from amazing schools around the world.

In 1999, she opened a school that became accredited in the holistic arts and ran that until 2012 teaching students from all over the world how to heal themselves and others.

The art of healing seems to open a gate to quantum energy, where magic seems to be taking place. But it must be a science since if I can teach others to do what I can do, it can't be just magic... and if these teachable gifts are in the Bible, then it has been teachable for over two thousand years.

Constance continually strives to advance her knowledge and is currently in the process of attaining her Ph.D. and DOCTORATE in Natural and Integrative Medicine.

ALSO AVAILABLE

Play the game *Ikona* – Discover Your Inner Genie

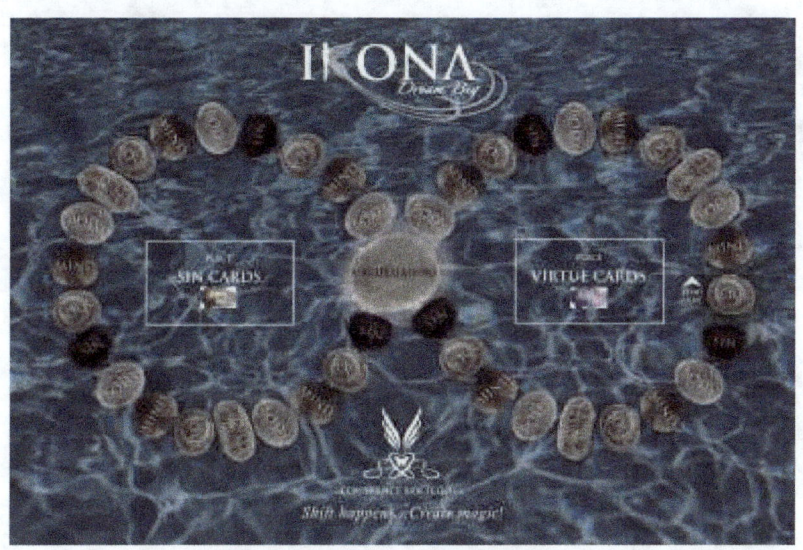

For additional information on

Constance Santego's

wide range of Motivational Products, Coaching Sessions,
Spiritual Retreats,
Live Events and Educational Programs

Go to

www.ConstanceSantego.ca

Follow on Instagram - Constance_Santego and
Facebook - constancesantegoo

Subscribe and receive Free Information and Meditations
on my
YouTube Channel - Constance Santego

www.ingramcontent.com/pod-product-compliance
Lightning Source LLC
Chambersburg PA
CBHW071812080526
44589CB00012B/766